MW01119229

# The Complete Guide To Constipation Relief Naturally

## By Petra Ennis

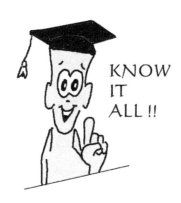

*To my husband Robert. Thank you for all your support.*

*My special thanks go to Gordon Smith for his help, good advice and editorial comments.*

# TABLE OF CONTENTS

## _Introduction_

I have written this book to give you the knowledge and tools to take charge of your health using natural methods for constipation relief.

As a Colonic Irrigation therapist I meet many people with digestive problems. I have patients who suffer with irritable bowel syndrome, diarrhoea, and flatulence but most of all I have patients suffering with constipation slight to severe symptoms.

I dedicated my spare time in the area of constipation research, I learned with practice and dedication natural methods to make my practice better and help hundreds of my patients.

Now I humbly present all of my research in this book to you so it can help your body restore bowel regularity, gain more health and digestive balance.

## *How to use this book*

Please keep in mind that this book is not a replacement of any of your doctor advice or prescriptions. For better results you may discuss any intended changes in your diet and life style with your doctor or your health practitioner.

In this book I will give you summary of diet advice, dietary supplements, healthy oils, herbs and herbal teas, folk remedies, food recipes, exercise tips and other useful hints on how to overcome constipation naturally.

As you will see for yourself there are plenty of ideas and valuable advice on what you can do to get rid of constipation. You will need to try a few of them and see what works for you as we are all different. You will not need to try every single food combination, herb or supplement.

Introduce life style changes slowly, and carefully. As you make changes watch diligently how your body and your bowel react.
Some changes may not agree with your system and you may need to try a different approach.

## Icons used in this Book

Pay attention, some important information for constipation relief.

Food, drink or habit which makes constipation worse.

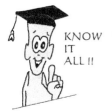

KNOW IT ALL !!  This little "Know it All" cartoon brings you broader information about health.

HOW TO USE ...  Explaining how to use massage oils, how to take supplements, how to prepare herbal teas etc., for achieving constipation relief.

WHERE ELSE TO FIND ...  Bring you information about foods containing important minerals and vitamins, which are necessary for a bowel to function properly.

# Chapter 1: Constipation

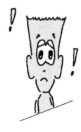 I believe that everyone had experienced difficulty passing stools at some point in their life. Some people occasionally, or chronically. But why is that and what can you do to avoid it? ...

## What is Constipation?

Constipation is difficulty passing stools.

It is a common digestive system problem in which a person has irregular bowel movements or passes hard stools or both. **It should not be ignored!**

**Bowel movements should be a regular every day event.** Healthy people should have two to three bowel movements a day. Having a bowel movement once a day is considered as slight constipation. Also, if it takes five minutes or more to complete a bowel movement, if you strain, or have pain or spasm during your time in the bathroom, then you have constipation.

A bowel movement should take no more than three minutes and requires very little toilet paper. It should leave your body easily with no discomfort. The stool should be mid-brown in colour, consistency of toothpaste, and quite long. There should be a mild smell or almost no smell.

## Is constipation dangerous?

Your colon (or large intestine) acts as a waste reservoir. It is the sewage plant of your body. It recycles the stuff your body can use (water, minerals, vitamins, etc.) and stores the rest for disposal. The waste lying in the colon is highly toxic. The colon wall is permeable which enables toxins to penetrate back into the body's blood stream. The longer waste sits in the colon, the longer **toxic materials** leach out of the solidifying stool into the blood. Blood toxins circulate through the whole body tissues, including all your organs and your brain.

**Many health issues can appear because of constipation. Some of them require a surgical treatment.**

Constipation influences your physical, emotional and mental wellbeing.

Examples of disorders which may be caused by constipation:

| | |
|---|---|
| abdomen distension | coated tongue |
| anal fissures | diabetes mellitus |
| appendicitis | diverticulitis |
| arthritis | depression |
| body odour | fatigue |
| bad breath | gas |
| bowel cancer | haemorrhoids |
| bowel polyps | headaches |
| Candida infection | hernia |

| | |
|---|---|
| indigestion | obesity |
| insomnia | prolapsus |
| lack of appetite | rheumatism |
| lethargy | skin problems |
| malabsorption | short memory loss |
| meningitis | thyroid disease |
| migraines | ulcerative colitis |
| myasthenia gravis | varicose veins |
| nervous exhaustion | |

*Constipation has an impact on your mood, energy levels, and sex life.*

Waste materials are not excreted only through the colon, but also through the **kidney**, **bladder**, **skin**, and **lungs**. If the colon does not work efficiently, the body will try to excrete increased toxins through these organs, which puts them under pressure. This may lead to some serious health problems. An example of this is chronic constipation and frequent urinary tract infections.

## *How the digestive organs work?*

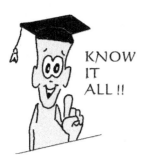

KNOW
IT
ALL !!

Our digestive tract is a long tube that is about nine metres/ thirty feet long in average.

Digestive process begins at the **mouth** where food is initially crushed and ground down by the teeth during chewing. The resulting ball, or "bolus", of food continues down the throat called **pharynx**, then travels through the gullet called **oesophagus** to the **stomach**, *small intestine*, *colon (or large intestine)*, *rectum* and *anus*. What cannot be digested in the stomach and small intestine is compacted as faeces in the colon and then eliminated.

Food travels through the system by a process of muscular contraction called *peristalsis*.

The digestive system is supported by glands (i.e. salivary gland), digestive organs such as the pancreas and liver. The pancreas and liver secrete *digestive juices* which help to break down the food in the stomach and small intestine.

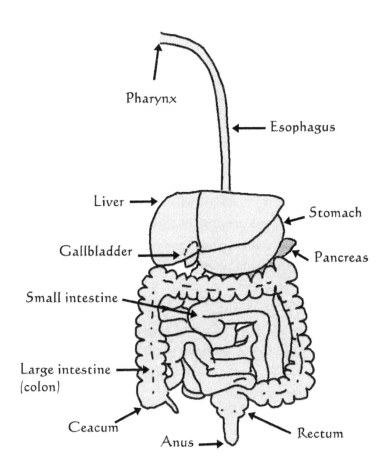

Once the waste reaches the first part of the colon – **Ceacum**, it looks like pea soup. It contains undigested food, water, some vitamins, salts and minerals. The waste continues its way into the **ascending colon, transverse colon, descending colon, sigmoid, rectum and anus**. During this journey; water is extracted from the waste and reabsorbed into the body. Vitamins and minerals are also absorbed. Faeces are then created.

**The whole digestive process can take up to 24 hours once everything works well.** It means that **we should have bowel movement once a day minimum!** If we have bowel movement twice or three times a day our digestion is working well.

It is very important that blood circulating in our body is clean and not polluted with dangerous toxins coming from a clogged up no-functioning colon.

Our lifestyle changed rapidly over the last few decades. It is much faster and more stressful. The air we breathe is polluted, the water we drink may contains chemicals (chlorine, fluorine compounds, hormones, nitrates, pesticides, trihalomethanes, salts of arsenic, radium, aluminium, copper, lead, mercury, cadmium, barium, ect.), the food we eat contains pesticides, preservatives, artificial colours, and other chemicals. Most of us lack exercise, we tend to solve our health problems with drugs like antibiotics and the list can go on and on. All these influence negatively on our digestive tract and are responsible for decreasing of friendly bacteria needed in our gut. Therefore we should make an effort and think before we put something into our mouth.

## *Causes of constipation*

There can be many causes of constipation.

Most people who suffer from constipation do not have a colon disorder. The problem usually lies in their eating and drinking habits.

### *Common reasons for constipation:*

- Dehydration
- Lack of natural fibre in the diet
- Nutritional deficiencies
- Excessive intake of protein and fat
- Too much cooked acid foods
- Certain beverages and foods consumed regularly, such as coffee, ordinary tea with milk, fizzy drinks, alcohol, tobacco, chocolate, sugar, etc.
- Eating unhygienic food
- Irregular eating habits
- Late night eating
- Magnesium and calcium deficiency
- Lack of exercise, physical activity
- Week abdominal muscles
- Stress, depression, emotional strain
- Busy lifestyle, not having time to "do my business"
- Travelling
- Irregular daily routine, shift work
- Ignoring the urge to have a bowel movement
- Build-up of faecal matter in the colon
- Mucus build-up in the colon
- Intestinal parasites, bad bacteria, infection, yeast infection (Candida)

- Medications, such as pain killers, antibiotics, blood pressure medications, heart medicines, antidepressants, antiparkinson drugs, diuretics, iron supplements, calcium supplements, antispasmodics, cough syrup and some antihistamines
- Some disorders such as anal fissure, amyloidosis, cancer, diabetes, hypocalcaemia, fibroids, intestinal obstruction, kidney failure, lupus, neurological disorders, metabolic and endocrine disorders, misaligned pelvis, multiple sclerosis, Parkinson's disease, scleroderma and systematic disorders, spinal cord injuries, stroke, thrombosed haemorrhoid, underactive or overactive thyroid gland, or uraemia
- Problems with hormonal control or with nerves and muscles in the colon, rectum, and anus
- Pregnancy

## Chapter 2: Food

 ### Food to avoid

***Food is often the main cause of constipation.***

The human digestive system was not designated to eat excessive amounts of meat, nor any refined foods like pizzas, hamburgers, chips, hot dogs, chocolate, ice cream, etc. which are commonly included in the modern diet. These types of food can cause harm to your body.

The food portions should be kept small. If you overeat, it puts the digestive organs under pressure which has a negative impact on other inner organs.

For healthier life style, and preventing constipation, *you should follow a low-fat diet, eat smaller portions and avoid heavy meals which are difficult to digest*. The last meal of the day should be at least three hours before bedtime. *Late night eating takeaway food and heavy dinners tend to cause constipation*.

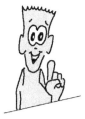

### *Avoid these foods as much as possible:*

- *Deep fry foods* such as potato chips and other types of take away foods.
- *Foods that stimulate excessive secretion of the mucous membranes*, such as dairy products (milk and cheese), fats, and spicy foods.
- Avoid *foods and drinks which are difficult to digest* and can irritate the intestinal lining such as:

| | |
|---|---|
| alcohol | milk |
| cakes | ordinary tea with milk |
| cheese | pastries |
| coffee | pizza |
| cookies | red meat |
| highly processed foods | salt |
| ice cream | soft drinks |

- Cut down or avoid **starchy foods** (such as potatoes, rice, bread, pasta) **as long as you are constipated** as eating them would only escalate the problem.
- Avoid **smoking**.

## Bread, Wheat and Gluten

**Gluten** is a composite of the proteins gliadin and glutenin, and is found in wheat, barley and rye. It is extremely resistant to intestinal digestion, despite grinding, cooking, and processing.

Most bread is made from wheat flour which contains protein Gluten. **Gluten can cause damage to the intestinal lining by eroding the villi and microvilli essential for digestion and absorption processes.**

Gluten intolerance symptoms:

| | | |
|---|---|---|
| anxiety | depression | migraines |
| acne and boils | diarrhoea | psoriasis |
| arthritis | eczema | skin rashes |
| bloating | flatulence | stomach pains |
| constipation | gas | tiredness |
| cramps | headaches | sweating, etc. |

Avoiding Gluten can improve your bowel movements in just few weeks; also you may lose excessive weight if desired.

If you become allergic to gluten and continue to eat gluten, you may develop celiac disease.

## Milk, Cheese and other Dairy Products

Dairy products contain a protein called **Casein**. Casein has large molecules which are hard to digest. This can cause irritation to the body and digestive tract and leads to excess mucus excretion.

*Dairy products are considered to be the most mucus forming foods.*

Eating dairy can lead to lung congestion, sinus congestion, and sticky constipated stools.

Dairy products also contain the sugar **Lactose**. In many cases the body is unable to break down the sugar Lactose because of enzyme Lactase deficiency. **Lactose intolerance leads to abdominal audible bowel sounds, bloating, constipation, cramps, diarrhoea, flatulence, and nausea.**

> If you suffer from constipation avoiding dairy products is highly recommended. Replace cow's milk with rice milk or almond milk.

## What to eat?

Once you avoid so many types of foods what should you eat instead?

- Your diet should consist mostly of **vegetables, fruits, sprouts, nuts and seeds, and grains**. Many people may think that vegetable dishes are plain but that is not true. There are many

13

vegetarian cook books out there with thousands of ideas for vegetable dishes which are delicious. It will maybe take a little bit of effort to find new recipes and change the diet habits but it is definitely worth it!

- Eat **lots of fruits;** they are slightly laxative and very beneficial for constipation relief. Avoid bananas and jack fruit.

- Switch to **gluten free bread.** You can find gluten free bread in your health store and in some supermarkets. Avoid wheat bread.

- **Try rice and almond milk, or goat milk and goat cheese instead of cow milk and cow cheese**. Also avoid soya milk and soya products as they may create hormonal imbalance.

- **Use honey or maple syrup** instead of sugar and sweeteners.

- Try **herbal teas instead of ordinary black tea with milk.**

- Instead of having sweets, have a piece of fruit or make a fruit cocktail for yourself and your family.

Eat when you are hungry, eat slowly, do not overeat, appreciate your food and never eat on the run or while watching television or working on your computer. Concentrate on your food and chew thoughtfully.

Do not forget to drink plenty of water, vegetable and fruit juices with no added sugar or sweeteners.

## _Why fibre is important in our diet?_

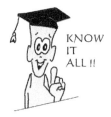

_The main function of fibre is to help maintain the healthy digestive tract. It speeds up excretion of the waste and toxins, preventing them from sitting in your colon for too long._

Fibre comes from plant's cell walls and we can get fibre only from plant based foods or from fibre powder products that you add to water and drink.

_There is no fibre in any meat, fish, eggs or dairy products._

Fibre is not a nutrient. It cannot be absorbed in the body and contains no calories or vitamins. It simply passes throw digestive system and comes out in the stool.

There are two types of fibre- _Insoluble and Soluble._
Both of them pass throw the digestive system unchanged until they reach the large intestine.

Insoluble fibre absorbs water, expands and creates a combination of bulk liquid in the colon. Stools then become soft and bulky which makes them travel through the colon more efficiently. In relation to this, insoluble fibre _reduces constipation and bowel diseases_ as toxins are absorbed by the fibre and leave the system.
Insoluble fibre can be found for example in beans, bran, brown rice, fruits, maize, oats, pulses, seeds, and whole grains.

Soluble fibre dissolves in water creating thick gel like substance which softens the stool. Soluble fibre can be found for example in apples, barley, citrus fruits, legumes, oats, pears, and strawberries.

Fibre brings enzymes to the colon which supports the growth of friendly gut bacteria, helps to get rid of old waste, keeps the colon flexible and strengthen the colon wall.

 *Include plenty of vegetable, fruits, seeds, nuts and grains in your diet.*

# Chapter 3: What influences bowel movements?

### Not having time to "do my business"

This is a very common factor which can lead to constipation. Our life style became so busy that often we do not have time to spend a few moments in the bathroom. Most people have their bowel movements in the morning before or shortly after breakfast. If you are already stressed in the morning, thinking about catching the bus or train to work or running around thinking about what you have to do during the busy day, the body releases **stress hormones which shut off bowel movements.** This is a major contributing factor in constipation.

If you have to work without **regular breaks** or have to do **shift work**, the colon may become irregular due to hormonal imbalances caused by shift work.

**Travelling** may also influence bowel movements. If you already know you may have a problem with constipation while you travel, get ready beforehand. Here are some useful tips:

- **Increase your fibre intake.** You may start a few days before your travel. The colon will be more prepared for changes this way. Add into your diet more **flaxseeds, nuts, fresh vegetables and fruits.**

- **Drink plenty of water and fresh made juices** (not from concentrate). Make it a habit to **carry a water bottle with**

17

*you on your travels* and make sure you drink at least three to four pints/two litres of water a day.

- Don't forget to **eat good healthy food**. When travelling many people tend to rush to the first fast food restaurant to acquire a burger or pizza, or rely heavily on cafe shops with a big selection of muffins and donuts. Definitely not the best solution!

- If you know you will be busy on your journey **prepare your lunch box and snacks beforehand**. There is nothing easier. It takes just few minutes and you will get a proper meal full of nutrients.

> **What can be in your lunch box?**
> Salad, fruit salad, oat crackers, chopped red or yellow pepper, cucumber sticks or celery sticks with hummus or any other healthy dip, bag of dried fruit or nuts, etc.

- **Do not forget to "move".** When travelling on business or on a busy mode of doing things, find few spare minutes in the morning or afternoon to perform some yoga postures in your hotel room or go for walk. Many hotels have gym of small swimming pool. There is always some way to exercise. **Exercise encourages bowel movements.**

## Excessive stress, worry, fear and grief cause constipation

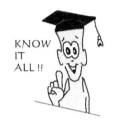

*..a few words about our nervous system...*

Human nervous system consists of **Central nervous system** (brain and spinal cord) and **Peripheral nervous system** (Cranial and Peripheral nerves). Peripheral nervous system consists of **Somatic nervous system** (voluntary control of body movements i.e. moving a finger) and **Autonomic nervous system** (responsible for control of involuntary or visceral bodily functions i.e. **digesting food**).

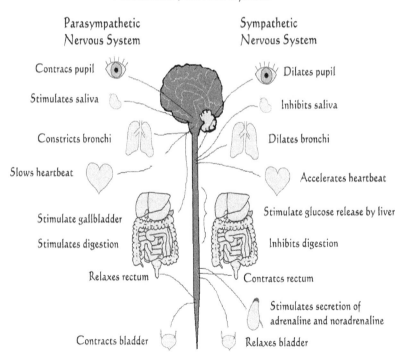

Autonomic Nervous System

Parasympathetic Nervous System — Sympathetic Nervous System

Contracs pupil — Dilates pupil
Stimulates saliva — Inhibits saliva
Constricts bronchi — Dilates bronchi
Slows heartbeat — Accelerates heartbeat
Stimulate gallbladder — Stimulate glucose release by liver
Stimulates digestion — Inhibits digestion
Relaxes rectum — Contratcs rectum
— Stimulates secretion of adrenaline and noradrenaline
Contracts bladder — Relaxes bladder

The **Autonomic nervous system controls _digestion_**, diameter of the pupils, heart rate, perspiration, respiration rate, salivation, sexual arousal and urination. Also, this system consists of the **Parasympathetic nervous system** (controls vegetative functions) and **Sympathetic nervous system (_allows body to function under STRESS_**, fight or flight response).**Only one of these systems can work at a time.**

On the picture with the Autonomic nervous system (page 19) you can see that the **digestive system is shut down while one is stressed.**

> Excessive stress can cause **constipation, diarrhoea, IBS, bloating, undigested food in the stool, etc.**

## Digestive juices

Digestive juices are produced by liver, pancreas and stomach glands. They are very important for proper digestion.

If the body is not able to release enough digestive juices from whatever reason, food in the stomach can start fragmenting and create gas. Abdominal discomfort, feeling sluggish, gas and pains can be the result. Lacking digestive juices also influences bowel movements.

- **Take your time** while eating. **Chew slowly** and put your attention on your meal.

Usually most people eat too fast and chew too little. Once you eat quickly and in a rush, or while you watch television or working on a computer, digestive juices are not released fully and digestive process cannot take place sufficiently.

Digestion is much easier task for the body once the food has been eaten slowly and properly broken down by chewing.

* If you eat slowly and still feel heavy, sluggish and bloated after every single meal, then your digestive organs may not be able to deliver enough digestive juices and enzymes. In this case you can boost your digestive juices with *digestive enzymes supplements*. You can find them in your pharmacy or health store. Follow the instruction on the label.

## Water Intake

Without proper hydration the faeces in the colon become very dry. This makes it harder for the colon to pass them thought its length and as a result constipation can occur.

* Drink, drink, drink - water is the key here. We should drink at about 3-4 pints/1.5-2 litres of water a day.

Coffee and ordinary black tea with milk (or without) is dehydrating. It can be a bit confusing as coffee and tea are liquids too, but unfortunately for coffee and black tea lovers they have dehydrating qualities.

## Muscular colon contractions – peristalsis

The waste in the colon can move through its length because of muscle contractions called peristalsis.

These contractions come in waves. If the muscle works properly the colon eliminates the waste smoothly.

In some cases nerves in the colon wall can be damaged by bad diet, lack of exercise or excessive use of laxatives. Therefore peristalsis cannot be performed properly and this can lead to *"lazy bowel syndrome" and constipation.*

- *Exercise*. Exercise stimulates peristalses and helps the waste to "move" through the colon.

- *Replace laxatives*. Laxatives weaken the nervous system in the colon wall and eventually make constipation even worse. Instead of laxatives use some type of natural colon cleanse. Example of good colon cleanse product is "Oxy-powder". This is a good natural colon cleanser which does not irritate or damage the intestinal lining. You can find plenty of similar products on the market.

## Laxatives

Laxatives are harsh and irritating to the bowel and they are not a long term solution for constipation relief.

Laxatives can bring a quick relieve from constipation but they can also be very harmful for the body. Laxatives weaken the nervous system of the colon wall which over time increases constipation. With excessive use you may develop a colon disorder called *"lazy bowel syndrome"* or *"atonic colon"*. With this disorder it is almost impossible to empty the bowel without taking some kind of laxatives.

Long term or excessive use of laxatives may also slow down your metabolism which eventually can lead to **nutritional deficiencies or malabsorption of nutrients from your food.**

Common side effects of using laxatives are:

| | |
|---|---|
| cramps | malabsorption |
| bloating and gas | spasms |
| diarrhoea | swollen abdomen |
| excessive thirst | weakness |
| lazy bowel syndrome | |

More serious side effects are:

| | |
|---|---|
| burning on urination | eyes problems |
| breathing difficulty | gastrointestinal blockage |
| confusion | irregular heartbeat |
| dizziness | irritability |
| difficulty swallowing | paralysis |
| ears and nose problems | rash and skin itching |

# Chapter 4: What to do to relieve constipation

 **_Drink plenty of water, pure fruit and vegetable juices_**

Dehydration is a far bigger problem than most people realize. It has an impact on the digestion, bowel movements and also on the general health and wellbeing.

When the waste reaches the caecum (the beginning of the colon) it contains lots of water. Most of this water is extracted from the waste and reabsorbed into the body. Faeces are then created.

If you do not drink enough liquids, faeces in the colon become very dry. This makes it difficult for the colon to pass them through its length. Also the mucous lining on the colon wall changes its consistency. It becomes thicker, failing to provide a slick lubricant for the movement of faeces.

It is recommended to drink a minimum of 3 pints/1.5 litres of water a day.

- **_Avoid dehydration at all costs_** and make a habit of drinking water all through the day. Do not drink flavoured water made from artificial sweeteners.
- Make a habit to start your day with a big glass of **_warm water with freshly squeezed lemon juice_** from half a lemon. It aids the digestive system and makes the process of eliminating wastes from the body easier.
- Drink **_purified room temperature or warm water_**. Ice-cold water gives a shock to the internal organs.

- For quick relief of constipation, drink a large glass of filtrated water every ten minutes for half an hour. This can work wonders to flush toxins out and relieve constipation.

- Try **Lemon and Honey Drink**

*Mix juice of half a lemon with one teaspoon of honey in the big glass of warm water. Drink one glass in the morning and one glass in the evening.*

Some people may experience tooth sensitivity after drinking lemon juice water (the acid the lemon juice carries may interfere with the tooth enamel). If you are one of them try lime and honey or just clear honey with warm water for your morning drink and skip the lemon juice.

Honey is a natural medicine and has plenty of benefits. One of them is **relieving constipation**.


## Squatting position

> **Nature designed the human body to eliminate waste in the squatting position.** The modern toilet makes our job harder because we are not in the correct position (i.e. squatting).

Once sitting on the toilet, the lower end of descending colon is bent, which requires a major muscular effort to evacuate the waste from the bowel. Once you strain, the little capillaries in the anal area can burst causing haemorrhoids.

*In the squatting position the colon aligns itself naturally with the rectum and anus which opens naturally and easily.*

25

There are **receptors on our calves** and once they are stimulated during squatting they relax the rectum muscles.

In the squatting position a person eliminates the stress and strain. This helps to prevent haemorrhoids, bloating and constipation as the transit time is reduced. One is able to pass much more faeces.

A little stool or step under your feet once you sit on the toilet may be a solution. This will bring your legs closer to the chest and with the slight leaning forward the squatting position is simulated.

You can buy a step specially designed for toilet use (see picture on the right), or you can use anything you have at home which would support your feet and bring your legs higher so you are in the squatting position. Once you have positioned  your feet on the step, relax, lean forward and place your elbows on your thighs.

 **Never ignore the urge to have a bowel movement** as the urge will disappear. Repeated ignoring of an urge will change the normal sensation in the rectum which can lead to constipation.

## Train your body

Try to have a bowel movement at the **same time every day**. The activity of the colon increases after waking up in the morning and after having your first meal. The urge to have a bowel movement is usually greatest after breakfast in most people.

Get up early enough in the morning to exercise (go for brisk walk or do some yoga postures), have breakfast, and sit on the toilet.

**Have patience**, it can sometimes take about 20 minutes to have a bowel movement. It also takes time to retrain your rectum muscles.

 ## Enemas

People have been using Enemas for centuries for constipation relief, gas relief, intestinal discomfort relief and to detox.

The use of an Enema is one of the quickest ways to relieve constipation. It is much better than taking laxatives or straining on the toilet for ages.

### What is an enema bag and how can you use it?

An enema bag is a plastic container (usually with the capacity of 4 pints/2 litres) with the thin hollow tube connected to it.

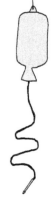

Fill the container with filtrated body temperature water and place it on the hook at about 4.5 - 5.5 feet/ 1.40 - 1.70 meters from the ground. Lie down on your back or your left side and insert the lubricated end of the tube into your anus and rectum. On the tube is a small valve you can regulate the water flow with. Introduce water slowly into your colon. Water will break down the hard stool and help faeces to move out of your colon.

**Very easy, very effective and can be used whenever is needed!**

You can also make herbal enemas, organic coffee or probiotic enemas for yourself as they are beneficial too, especially for detox purposes and for restoring good gut bacteria.

Contraindications for Enemas – see bottom of this page

 ## Colonic Irrigation/Hydrotherapy

**Colonic irrigation** is a kind of advanced enema. The difference between an enema and colonic irrigation is that **colonic irrigation washes out the whole length of the colon**, classic enema only washes out the sigmoid and descending part of the colon. That's only about 50% of the colon.

KNOW IT ALL !!

**Colon Irrigation is very effective for constipation relief.**

**If you suffer with severe constipation a number of colonics are usually needed.**

Colonic Irrigation cannot be done at home. You need to find a good clinic with a good colonic irrigation therapist. Experienced therapist will tell you how many colonics you will need after your first visit. The therapist should also discuss your diet with you and recommend some diet changes, food supplements, etc. if needed.

Contraindications for Colonics and Enemas
Abdominal hernia, active fistulas and fissures, aneurysm, carcinoma of the colon, cirrhosis of the liver, Chron's disease, colon cancer, diverticulitis, epilepsy or psychoses, gastrointestinal haemorrhage or perforation, high blood pressure not controlled by

a doctor, kidney failure, pregnancy, recent abdominal surgery, recent colorectal surgery, recent heart attack, rectal or abdominal tumours, severe anaemia, severe cardiac disease, ulcerative colitis.

In the case of any intestinal disorder consult your doctor or your health practitioner.

 ## Complementary/Holistic Therapy

Therapies that can treat constipation are **Acupressure, Acupuncture, Ayurvedic Medicine, Chinese Herbal Medicine, Homeopathy, and Herbalism**.

In some cases constipation can be caused by sacrum injury, pelvis misalignment, body energy imbalance, or shock persisting in the body causing the harm. In these cases try **Cranio-Sacral Therapy** (good for fixing sacrum injury, pelvis misalignment and other energetic issues in your body)**, Cranial Osteopathy, Osteopathy, Kinesiology, and Chiropractic or Visceral manipulation**.

Always make sure your complementary/ holistic therapy practitioner is properly trained and well experienced!

 ## Self - abdominal Massage

Massaging of the abdominal area regularly will strengthen muscles of the colon wall and improve peristalsis (the wave like movement of the colon muscle). The gentle pressure applied on the colon helps to loosen the stool and to move it towards the rectum.

*The massage technique:*

Start on the lower right side of your abdomen area. This is where the ileocecal valve, cecum and appendix are. The movements of your hand should be circular and clockwise. Move your hand slowly upwards towards your ribcage. Once your hand reaches the first rib on your ribcage continue to your left across your abdomen following the transverse colon. Once you are on the left side of your abdomen move downwards towards your groin. Waste matter flows in this direction.

Start with gentle pressure and increase the pressure after a few days. Use massage oils for better results.

Perform abdominal massage 3-4 times a day for 5 minutes.

Slight pain can be experienced on the beginning of the massage. This happens usually in the case of severe constipation or if you suffer from flatulence. This pain should ease during the massage or completely disappear.

*If you feel deep pain in your colon area, stop the massage. If the pain persists contact your doctor or your health care practitioner.*

 **Supplements**

There are some specific supplements which can be beneficial to take when you are constipated.

*If you are on any medication or suffer from any kind of disease or disorder (kidney disease, liver disease, heart disorder, etc.) consult your doctor or your health care practitioner before taking supplements.*

### Magnesium

Many people who suffer from constipation are lacking magnesium.

Magnesium causes movement of fluid into the bowel which makes faeces softer and helps with bowel movements. Magnesium relaxes muscles of the colon wall allowing for a normal peristaltic action.

HOW TO USE ...

*Take 400 – 1,000mg Magnesium daily before bedtime. The dose for magnesium is individual. Start with the lower dosage 400mg a day and increase as needed. If you experience loose stool, reduce the dosage.*

WHERE ELSE TO FIND ...

Foods rich in magnesium include apples, apricots, avocados, bananas (avoid bananas if you suffer with constipation), berries, blackstrap molasses, brown rice, cabbage, cantaloupe, cornmeal, dulse, figs, garlic, grains, grapefruit, green leafy vegetables, honey, kelp, lemons, lima beans, millet, nuts, peaches, pears, black-eyed peas, prunes, sesame seeds, soybeans, spinach, watercress, and whole grains.

### Calcium

Calcium works with magnesium to regulate the muscle tone.

HOW TO USE ...

*Take 700 - 1,100mg daily. It is necessary to take Calcium and Magnesium supplements together as Calcium supplements taken on their own can cause constipation.*

WHERE ELSE TO FIND ...

Calcium is found in dark green leafy vegetables, almonds, asparagus, broccoli, cabbage, cauliflower, carob, celery, collards, dandelion greens, dulse, figs,

31

filberts, kale, kelp, lemon, mustard greens, oats, prunes, rhubarb, sesame seeds, soybeans, turnip greens, watercress, and whey.

## Probiotics

Probiotics are live microbial organisms that are naturally present in the digestive tract.

They are vital for proper digestion, and also perform a number of other useful functions such as preventing the overgrowth of the yeast bacteria (Candida) and other pathogens, and synthesizing vitamin K.

HOW TO USE ...

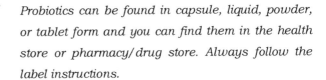

*Probiotics can be found in capsule, liquid, powder, or tablet form and you can find them in the health store or pharmacy/drug store. Always follow the label instructions.*

The imbalance of the intestinal flora and lack of good bacteria can lead to digestive problems such as constipation, diarrhoea, Irritable Bowel Syndrome (IBS), ulcerative colitis, Crohn's disease, pouchitis, bad bacterial overgrowth, Candida, and vaginal yeast infections.

We can disturb intestinal flora by taking medications (such as antibiotics), an unhealthy diet with inadequate dietary fibre intake, busy lifestyle, or ingestion of environmental toxins (smoking/alcohol/Drugs).

WHERE ELSE TO FIND ... Food rich in probiotics are buttermilk, kefir, miso, sauerkraut, tempeh, umeboshi, and probiotic yogurt.

### Aloe Vera Juice

Aloe Vera is anti-inflammatory, anti-bacterial and anti-viral.

It has the potential to soothe irritations in the digestive tract, such as ulcers, colitis, Irritable Bowel Syndrome, or bloating. **Aloe Vera aids in forming soft stools encouraging daily regularity.** The juice also actively encourages the release of gastric enzyme pepsin which is necessary for the digestive process.

HOW TO USE ...  *Follow the label instruction.*
*Aloe Vera Juice can be diluted in the glass of water or juice.*

Aloe Vera will help you repair damaged tissue in the intestines and stimulates all of the digestive glands, stomach, kidneys, gallbladder and liver to function properly.

### Oxy-Powder

Oxy-Powder is one of the best Natural colon cleansers on the market today. It is **natural**, and comparing to laxatives, it would not do any harm to intestines.

HOW TO USE ...  *Oxy-Powder can be taken for one week colon cleanse or whenever is needed instead of laxatives. Follow the label instruction.*

### Fruit, vegetable, and grain Supplement (FVGS)

FVGS provides whole food nutrition from many different fruits, vegetables, and grains in the capsule form. This supplement has plenty of health benefits including constipation relief.

33

*Follow the label instruction.*

### Triphala

Triphala is originally Indian herbal blend, which has been found to act as a complete body cleanser. It is one of the most commonly used herbal blends in Ayurvedic medicine.

HOW TO USE ... 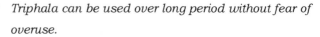 *Triphala can be used over long period without fear of overuse.*

*Follow the label instruction.*

### Kyolic Garlic

Kyolic Garlic is an aged garlic product usually in capsules. Aging garlic is a stronger more stable product, and less irritable to the digestive system with no garlic odour.

HOW TO USE ...

 *Take 6 Kyolic capsules just before bedtime.*

Kyolic Garlic is a great aid for digestive problems, improves bowel movements, helps to kill bad bacteria and fungus in the digestive tract including Candida infection, and it has cleansing properties.

### Psyllium Husks

Psyllium Husk is well proven supplement which helps digestive tract by removing waste from the bowel. However, if you suffer by severe constipation you should not consider taking this supplement as in some cases Psyllium Husks can make your constipation worse.

34

Psyllium Husks expanse in the bowel. If you do not drink enough water, Psyllium may create a blockage in your bowel.

HOW TO USE ... *In the case of mild constipation mix 2 tablespoons of Psyllium Husks in a glass of water and drink immediately. Follow with another glass or two of water or juice. Psyllium Husks should be taken in the morning and in the evening half an hour before or after meals.*

*If you do not drink enough water do not take Psyllium Husks.*

## Lubrication of the digestive tract

Healthy Oils are cold pressed plant based oils, known sometimes also as virgin oils. They are high in important fatty acids, minerals and nutrients, which our body needs for proper functioning, as opposed to animal based fats which can be harmful to the human body.

Cold pressed oils can be used on a daily basis. These oils speed up fat metabolism, hence they are not fattening when used in moderation.

> By using the healthy Oils the digestive tract becomes more lubricated. This improves digestion and prevents/relieves constipation.

HOW TO USE ... *Cold pressed oils are great in salads, soups (pour a little bit of oil into your soup just before serving),* smoothies or juices. Cold pressed oil can be spread on a piece of non-wheat bread instead of butter or margarine, or can be used for making pesto or dips.

**Cold pressed oils should not be boiled or used for frying (except coconut oil) as its important components would be destroyed and turn rancid.**

### Flaxseed Oil

Flaxseed Oil is considered to be nature's richest source of omega-3 fatty acids. It also contains omega 6 and omega-9 fatty acids, lecithin, magnesium, potassium, zinc, and B vitamins.

HOW TO USE ...

*Take 1-2 tablespoonfuls of Flaxseed Oil daily with lots of water right after your lunch or dinner.*

*Flaxseed Oil can be also mixed in the glass of apple juice or in a smoothie.*

*Include Flaxseed Oil in your homemade salad dressings.*

### Extra Virgin Olive Oil

Extra Virgin Olive Oil is a concentrated source of monounsaturated fats, polyphenolic phytonutrients that have antioxidant activity, vegetable mucilage and antioxidant vitamin E.

There are many types of olive oils (Virgin Olive Oil, Pure Olive Oil, etc.), but Extra Virgin Olive Oil is considered the best, least processed, comprising of oil from the first pressing of the olives. Extra Virgin Olive Oil is the best quality Olive Oil.

Use Extra Virgin Olive Oil in your salad dressings, pour a little bit of Extra Virgin Olive Oil into your soups just before serving, drizzle over your vegetable dishes, use in dips or spread on piece of non-wheat bread instead of butter.

Mix 1 teaspoonful of Extra Virgin Olive Oil with fresh lemon juice squeezed from ½ a lemon. Drink in the morning on an empty stomach.

Mix ¼ cup of Extra Virgin Olive Oil with ½ cup of apple or orange juice and drink (it has a unsavoury taste but improves constipation relief). Have this drink once a week preferably in the evening time.

### Extra Virgin Coconut Oil

Extra Virgin Coconut Oil is considered one of nature's highest sources of medium chain fatty acids and saturated fats.

HOW TO USE ...  Use Extra Virgin Coconut Oil in salads dressings. Add ½ teaspoon of Extra Virgin Coconut Oil into your fruit and vegetable smoothie.

**Coconut Oil can be used daily for baking and cooking instead of other oils. Heating does not harm this oil.**

### Extra Virgin Avocado Oil

Extra Virgin Avocado Oil is rich in monounsaturated fatty

acids, vitamin A, B group vitamins, vitamin D and E, sterols, lecithin, lutein, alpha and beta carotene, and other essential fatty acids.

HOW TO USE ...

*Take 2-4 tablespoonfuls of Avocado Oil daily for constipation relief.*

*Drizzle Extra Virgin Avocado Oil over your salads, soups, vegetable dishes, seafood dishes, use in guacamole or other dips, or use as bread spread.*

*You can also mix Avocado Oil with apple or orange juice and drink.*

### Almond Oil

Almond Oil is rich in essential fatty acids, vitamin A, B group vitamins, vitamin E and D, and other important minerals.

HOW TO USE ...

*Take 2-4 tablespoons of Almond Oil daily for constipation relief.*

*Use Almond oils for making your salad dressings, use in dips, as a bread spread or drizzle over your vegetable and seafood dishes.*

Other types of Oil which can be used in the diet for constipation relieve are: **Canola oil, Garlic oil, Grapeseed oil, Pumpkin oil, Safflower oil, and Sesame oil.**

It is also possible to take Omega 3 supplements for relieving constipation, but if you include Healthy Oils regularly in your diet there is no need for them. Better to develop healthy eating habits instead of relying on nutrient capsules or supplements.

 ## *Natural Foods with Mild Laxative Properties*

What should you include in your diet once you suffer from constipation?

**_Apple_** – Apples are one of the most cultivated fruit.
Apples are rich in fibre, they add bulk to the stool, thus help digestion, constipation relieve and digestive disorders.

- *Have 3-4 ripe apples a day as a healthy snack or add them into your fruit salads, smoothies and juices.*
- *Buy organic apples and do not peel the skin.*

Some people may experience bloating and gas after eating an apple. In this case the apple was not ripe enough or you may have developed food intolerance to apples.
If you get bloated every single time after eating an apple, eat apples in moderation or avoid them completely.

**_Apple Cider Vinegar_** - Apple cider vinegar is made from fresh ripe apples that are fermented.
Apple cider vinegar helps the body in performing natural bowel movements. It contains significant amounts of pectin, which is a water soluble fiber that helps to improve digestion by normalizing the acid levels in the stomach.

- *Mix 2-3 teaspoons of Apple Cider Vinegar in 200 ml of water. Drink this mixture three times a day before meal. If required use apple juice or grape juice instead of water for better taste.*

**Bael Fruit** – Bael Fruit has been cultivated in India for over 4,000 years and is highly valued for its perceived medicinal qualities especially in Ayurvedic practise.
Bael Fruit cleans and tones up the intestines and its regular use for two or three months helps to remove the old accumulated faecal matter from the bowels.

- *Have about 2-2.3 oz (60-70 grams) of the Bael Fruit a day preferably before dinner*
- *Bael Fruit can be taken with honey to make it more palatable*

**Beetroot** - Beetroot helps stimulate the bowels, thus helps relieve constipation.

- *Have two small raw beetroots in the morning time as a healthy snack.*
- *Include the beetroots is your salads*
- *You may also cook the beetroots and serve in various vegetable dishes.*
- *Use mainly raw beetroots for constipation relief, cook just occasionally.*

*There is a special way how to cook beetroots.*
Before cooking beets, cut one inch off the tops. This helps lock in the nutrients during cooking and you will not lose them.

40

Beetroots should be cooked whole and then peeled; otherwise, they bleed all their colour and nutrients into the water.

**Cantaloupe** – Cantaloupe is the most popular variety of melon. Cantaloupe is one of the easiest foods to digest, it is sweet and cooling. It is packed with fibre, thus helps with bowel movements, relieves constipation and reduces stomach gas.

- *Include a Cantaloupe in your fruit salads or eat it on its own as a healthy snack.*
- *Add a Cantaloupe into your fruit smoothies and fruit juices.*

**Cabbage** – Cabbage has been used in the kitchen for centuries and is one of the oldest dishes in history. It has wonderful cleansing properties in the stomach and the intestines.

- *For constipation relief, cabbage should be eaten raw or it can be juiced. Raw cabbage is more easily digested then the cooked one.*
- *Have a cabbage salad for your lunch or dinner twice a week*
- *Include the cabbage in your vegetable salads or use cabbage as a side dish.*
- *Juice the cabbage and drink two glasses of cabbage juice a day.*
- *Make a cabbage soup once or twice a week.*
- *Use cabbage in your stir-fries.*

If you decide to cook the cabbage, blanch the quartered cabbage for 5-10 minutes, then discharge the water and continue cooking in fresh water. In this case you may avoid gas after eating it.

**Cucumber** – cucumber is a widely cultivated plant. Cucumber is a laxative food. It supplies bulk to the stool, helps to promote the flexibility of colon cells and supports bowel regularity.

- *Include the cucumber in your salads.*
- *Use the cucumber as a dipping stick instead of breadstick (i.e. cut cucumber into 5 cm long sticks and use hummus as a dip).*
- *Eat ½ or 1 small cucumber as a healthy snack.*
- *Drink 1-2 glasses of fresh cucumber juice daily.*

*Cucumber juice tips:*
- Juice 1 large cucumber, 2cm piece fresh ginger root, add ½ cup of water and serve immediately.
- Juice 1 cucumber, ½ watermelon, add ½ cup of water and serve immediately.
- Juice 1 cucumber, 5 carrots, 1 beetroot, add 1 cup of water and serve immediately.
- Juice 1 cucumber, 5 apples, 6 celery sticks and serve immediately.

**Dates** – Dates are high in fibre which helps to clear the digestive tract and aid intestinal disturbances.

- *Dates should be immersed in water overnight before eating to secure laxative effect. Soak 6 dates in hot water overnight, drink the water in the morning and eat the dates.*
- *Eat dried dates as a healthy snack during the day.*

**_Figs_** – Figs promote the healthy bowel function and prevent constipation due to the high levels of fibre.

- *Cut the dry figs into small pieces and add them to your home muesli or sprinkle them over your morning cereals.*
- *Have a handful of the dry or fresh figs as a healthy snack.*
- *Add the figs into your fresh vegetable and fruit salads.*

**_Garlic_** – Garlic is considered to be a superfood.

Garlic had been used in natural medicine for centuries for its healing qualities. Eating Garlic (raw or in the tablet form) assists the relief of constipation.

Garlic is rich in potassium which is essential for proper contractions of the muscles, including intestinal muscles. Garlic has an ability to cleanse and reduce inflammation throughout whole gastrointestinal tract. It kills bad bacteria and pathogens which at times appear in our insides, especially in the colon.

Garlic can be eaten raw or in capsule form (Kyolic Garlic capsules see page 34) to avoid the garlic odour.

Garlic can be also cooked in the different meals. The healing properties of the cooked garlic are much lower than healing properties of raw garlic.

- *Eat one or two raw gloves of garlic three times a day.*
- *Include raw chopped garlic in the salads, dips or bread spreads, or add minced raw garlic into your homemade soup just before serving.*

Raw and Kyolic Garlic are anti-flatulent. Cooked garlic may cause flatulence in some people.

**_Grapes_** - Grapes are a laxative food. They help to tone up the stomach and intestines.

- *Have a bunch of grapes (at least 350gm) every day*
- *You can also eat the dried grapes - Raisins. For constipation relief; soak raisins for at least twelve hours in the water and eat them preferably in the morning.*
- *Include grapes in your morning muesli.*
- *If grapes make you feel bloated eat them in moderation.*

**_Guava_** – Guava is a tropical fruit. It has a shape of pear, with green rind and pinkish or white flesh and small seeds.

- *Have one or two guavas every day as a healthy snack. Try to eat guava with seeds as it is more beneficial for constipation relief.*

**_Kiwi_** – Kiwi fruits stimulate and improve bowel movements. Daily intake of Kiwi fruit will lead to softer and bulkier faeces which improve excretion. Kiwis help to increase good bacteria in the digestive tract, strengthen the absorption ability of the intestine, and aids in the prevention of colon cancer.

- *For constipation relief consume three kiwis one hour before bedtime.*
- *If you are over 60 years of age consume two kiwis two hours before sleep.*
- *You can also have kiwi as a healthy snack during the day or add one kiwi or two into your fruit salads and smoothies.*

44

***Mango*** - Mango is cultivated in many tropical countries and distributed widely in the world.

Mango helps to soothe digestive problems such as constipation, indigestion, hyperacidity, flatulence, diarrhoea, dysentery, and haemorrhoids.

- *Include Mango in your fruit and vegetable salads, smoothies, juices or have it as a healthy snack. Mango is also good in the salad dressings.*
- *Consume one medium size mango a day or every second day.*

***Manuka Honey*** - Honey is a natural medicine. Manuka Honey is a special type of honey only found in the New Zealand. It has natural antibacterial, antimicrobial, antiviral, antiseptic, anti-inflammatory properties.

Manuka Honey is beneficial for maintaining a healthy digestive system as it helps intestines to function better. Manuka Honey helps constipation relief, aids poor digestion, Irritable Bowel Syndrome, and stomach ulcers as the honey coats and protects the stomach while it can fight the bacteria.

- *Have 1 full tablespoon of Manuka Honey every morning on an empty stomach or mix 1 teaspoon of Manuka Honey with 1 teaspoon of apple cider vinegar in a glass of water. Drink from 1-3 times a day.*

***Molasses*** - Molasses is a thick by-product from the processing of the sugar beet or sugar cane into sugar.

Blackstrap molasses aid constipation, cramping and digestive troubles.

- *Add 1 to 2 tablespoons a day to your breakfast cereals or mix with warm water, fruit juice or rice milk and drink slowly.*

**Oat Bran** - Due to its high level of dietary fibre oat bran aids digestion, helps relieve constipation, irritable bowel syndrome, diverticulitis, gastritis and lowers risk of bowel cancer.

- *Mix 1/3 cup of oat bran with your breakfast cereals every morning.*

**Orange** – Orange helps to stimulate digestive juices in the digestive tract, relieving constipation. Orange juice also excites peristaltic activity and helps prevent the accumulation of food residue in the colon. Orange helps to ease bowel disorders and indigestion.

- *Have two sweet oranges in the morning and two sweet oranges at bedtime.*

**Papaya** - Papaya contains papain, an enzyme that helps digest proteins. In fact, papain has been extracted to make dietary supplements for digestion.
Papaya aids digestion and thus prevents constipation.

- *Papaya should be eaten at breakfast time for it to act as a laxative.*
  *Have half a medium-sized papaya for breakfast in your breakfast fruit salad or add papaya to your morning smoothie.*

**_Pear_** – Pear is excellent source of water-soluble fibre. The pectin in pears is diuretic and has a mild laxative effect, thus helps to relieve constipation.

- *Add one medium sized pear into your morning fruit salad, cut one pear into small pieces and mix with your breakfast cereals, or include one pear in your morning smoothie.*
- *Have one pear after your dinner as a healthy snack.*
- *Drinking Pear Juice regularly help regulate bowel movements.*

*In some cases bloating may be experienced after having a pear. In this case consume the pears in moderation.*

**_Persimmon_** - Persimmon is a deep orange waxy fruit which is similar to a tomato in shape. This fruit is very popular in Japan China, and eastern US.

The raw Persimmon helps to treat constipation, diarrhoea, and haemorrhoids.

- *Have one or two Persimmons a day as a healthy snack or include a Persimmon in your fruit salads and smoothies*
- *Do not consume too many persimmons at once as they can induce diarrhoea.*

**_Pineapple_** – Pineapple is a delicious fruit cultivated in tropical countries. It contains a proteolytic enzyme called bromelain, which improves the digestion of protein.

Pineapple contains lots of fibre, hence it aids digestion, relieves stomach upsets, prevents and relieves constipation, and helps fight intestinal parasites.

- *Include a Pineapple in your fruit and vegetable salads, smoothies and juices.*
- *Consume a Pineapple on its own as a healthy snack before bed time.*

**Plums and Prunes** – Plums have a mild laxative effect. They are high in fibre which helps to cleanse the intestines, reduces gas and keeps the colon healthy.

Prunes are dried Plums. They contain much more fibre then Plums; they are more effective in treating constipation.

- *Have Plums or Prunes in the morning with your breakfast cereals, during the day as a healthy snack or before bedtime.*
- *Have 5 Plums or 10 Prunes a day.*

**Prune Juice** – Prune Juice is made by pressing prunes. It is one of the traditional remedies used for constipation relief. Prune Juice can be bought in every health store and in some supermarkets.

Prune juice promotes regularity by providing simple sugars that draw fluid into the intestine. The additional fluid makes a stool softer and easier to expel.

- *Have one glass of Prune Juice in the morning before your breakfast or in the evening before your bedtime every day for 10 days.*

Do not use prune juice on a long term basis as the intestines become dependent on it to function properly. Consuming too much of the juice can also result in kidney problems.

**_Raspberries_** – Raspberries improve digestion. Their small cellulose-rich "seeds" promote intestinal transit and effectively prevent constipation and stomach-ache.

- *Add Raspberries into your breakfast cereals and smoothies or have Raspberries during the day as a healthy snack.*

**_Rhubarb_** – Rhubarb has a mild laxative effect, it helps counterbalance stomach acid and thus, it is beneficial for those suffering from indigestion.

- *The best way is to eat Rhubarb raw on its own or in salads, or it can be added into fruit and vegetable juices and smoothies. Do not cook Rhubarb as it is high in oxalic acid and once cooked this acid is converted into inorganic chemical which can harm the body. Also never eat rhubarb leaves as they contain toxic chemicals.*

> **Rhubarb Juice**
> *4 apples*
> *2 Rhubarb stalks*
> *2 pears*
> Juice and drink 1-2 times a day

If you do not like taste of rhubarb or rhubarb juice you can get rhubarb supplements as a replacement from the health store. A well-known type is called Chinese rhubarb root which can be taken instead.

*If you have arthritis or gout, do not consume rhubarb.*

**Sauerkraut** – Sauerkraut is fermented food and it supplies the digestive tract with living cultures (Lactobacillus plantarum). This bacterium is a very dominant strain of healthful bacteria which helps digestive system by breaking down food and assimilating nutrients, and immune system by increasing antibodies that fight infectious disease.

Eating Sauerkraut is a great way to protect the balance of bacteria in the gastrointestinal tract. It is also beneficial to consume sauerkraut once one suffers by Candida (yeast) infection.

- *For constipation relief drink twice a day 250 ml glass of raw Sauerkraut juice. You may follow it by 250 ml glass of grapefruit juice for better results.*
- *Include Sauerkraut in your meals as a side dish or as a part of your salad dishes.*

**Spinach** – Raw spinach contains the finest organic material for the cleansing, reconstruction, and regeneration of the intestinal tract. Especially raw Spinach Juice is great cure for constipation.

- *Drink 250 ml glass of spinach juice first thing in the morning and last thing at night. You can dilute it with pure water. This drink should work wonders in just couple of days.*
- *Consume Spinach Salads regularly.*

 *Avoid spinach if you suffer from hepatitis, rheumatism, gastric and intestinal inflammations.*

### Nuts and Seeds

Nuts and seeds provide fibre and healthy oils. Consuming nuts and seeds soften and brakes down the stool which helps in excretion.

Nuts and seeds are also excellent sources of protein, minerals, healthy mono-unsaturated fats, other nutrients, and antioxidants.

**Stick to the raw and unsalted variety of nuts and seeds.**

To get the best from nuts and seeds, you should chew them well or grind them before eating.

Include in your diet these types of nuts: **Almonds, Brazil Nuts, Cashew Nuts, Pecan nuts, Walnuts, Hazelnuts, Chestnuts, Pine Nuts, Pistachios and Macadamias, Flaxseeds, Hemp Seeds, Sunflower Seeds, Pumpkin Seeds, and Sesame Seeds.**

HOW TO USE ... *Add nuts and seeds to your morning home-made muesli, sprinkle them over your vegetable and fruit salads, add them into various dishes, or eat them as a healthy snack.*

*Make a mixture of the seeds and nuts, and have it stored and ready to use.*

*Nuts are high in calories. Do not consume too much of them. Maximum should be around 25-50g of nuts a day.*

51

..a few words about **Flaxseeds**

Flaxseeds are very effective in relieving constipation and there are some special ways to use them.

HOW TO USE ...

*Grinding flaxseeds makes it easier for the body to reap the fibre and omega-3 fatty acid benefits.*

*Soak 1 tablespoon of flaxseeds in a glass of water overnight and drink this mixture twice a day.*

*Boil two cups of water with two tablespoons of flaxseed for fifteen minutes. Strain off the flaxseed, pour into a cup, add one teaspoon of apple cider vinegar and drink on an empty stomach. You can dilute this jelly like substance with a little bit of water if needed. Drink daily for 2 weeks.*

*Do not fry or heat flaxseeds. Chemical reactions involved in frying flaxseeds are harmful for your body.*

***Don't forget to drink plenty of water as flaxseeds suck liquids with toxins from your body.***

Sprout the seeds, nuts, legumes and grains. Sprouted seeds, nuts, legumes and grains are considered as the most enzyme-rich food on the planet. Beside the other health benefits these life enzymes help with ***digestion!***

**Spice & Herbs for Constipation Relief**

### Amla powder / Indian gooseberry

Amla powder is made from Amla fruit known as well as Indian gooseberry. All parts of the Amla plant are used in various Ayurvedic and herbal preparations.

HOW TO USE ...  *Mix 1 teaspoon of Amla powder and 1 teaspoon of honey in 200 ml of warm water. Drink on empty stomach or before bedtime.*

*Blend Amla powder in soups, salads, sauces, spicy foods, rice or gravies.*

*Do not take more than 2 teaspoons a day.*

### Asafoetida

Asafoetida is a spice native to Iran. It has been commonly used in Middle Eastern and Indian herbal medicine for digestive problems.

HOW TO USE ...  *Use Asafoetida in vegetarian and fish dishes. It goes very well with aubergines, baked potatoes, and is great in Indian "Dahl" which is cooked red lentils with spices.*

*Add Asafoetida into your soups, sauces and dips.*

### Basil

Basil, same as Ginger, has been used in traditional medicines for centuries for treating various health conditions.

HOW TO USE ...  *Use Basil in salads, soups, pesto, sauces or dips.*

*Make a Basil Tea by infusing 2 teaspoonfuls of dried basil leafs or 8 fresh basil leaves in 200ml of boiling water for 10 minutes. Strain before drinking.*

Avoid Basil during Pregnancy.

### Cardamom

Cardamom is native to the Middle East, North Africa, and Scandinavia. It can be found in many Indian sweet dishes. Cardamom is also commonly used in Ayurvedic medicine.

HOW TO USE ...

*Cardamom is nice in curries, lentils, rice dishes or vegan rice pudding.*

*For Cardamom Tea put 10 pulverized seeds into 500 ml of water, add 2 teaspoons of fresh grinded ginger and a cinnamon stick. Simmer for 15 minutes. Sweeten with honey. Drink 2-3 cups a day.*

### Cayenne Pepper

Many herbalists believe Cayenne is the most useful and valuable herb in the herb kingdom.

Cayenne is considered as a Superfood.

**Cayenne Pepper helps the entire body health and wellbeing.** It aids whole digestive system, improves peristaltic action of the intestines, hence it is great for constipation relief. Cayenne also reduces gas, spasms and abdominal cramping, helps to rebuild the tissue in the stomach, aids assimilation, supports digestive juices production, kills bad bacteria in digestive tract, prevents stomach ulcers formation, and is great for heartburn.

HOW TO USE ...

*Cayenne Pepper can be added into many dishes. Sprinkle Cayenne over your salads and soups; add Cayenne into the stir fries, curries, smoothies, etc.*

*Start your day with a 1/3 teaspoon of Cayenne Pepper in glass of warm water. Add fresh lemon juice and sweeten with honey if required.*

*You can also buy Cayenne Pepper capsules in your health store but try to use Cayenne Pepper in spicing your dishes first as taking Cayenne in meals or drinks is more beneficial.*

### Chickweed

Chickweed has established itself all over the world. It is very nutritious herb high in vitamins and minerals.

HOW TO USE ...

*Include Chickweed in your salads.*
*Chickweed is great in pesto, or it can be cooked as a pot herb.*
*For Chickweed tea infuse 1 tablespoon of dried or 3 tablespoons of fresh herb, add it into 200 ml boiling water and steep for 10 minutes. Drink 2 to 4 times a day.*

### Cinnamon

Cinnamon is found in most tropical countries and it is one of the oldest known spices.

HOW TO USE ...

*Use ground Cinnamon in smoothies and juices.*
*Sprinkle ground Cinnamon over your morning porridge or your morning cereals.*
*Sprinkle ground Cinnamon over your fruit salads.*
*For Cinnamon Tea break one cinnamon stick into pieces and place in a cup. Add 200 ml of boiling water and keep covered for 10-15 minutes. Stain*

*before drinking. If you like add honey and fresh lemon juice.*

*You can also place a cinnamon stick into any type of herbal tea to add flavour and health benefits.*

## Coriander

Coriander is commonly used around the world in the different cuisines. This herb is especially popular in India.

HOW TO USE ...   *Use Coriander in your kitchen for spicing your meals.*

## Cumin

Cumin is originally from Iran and the Mediterranean.

HOW TO USE ...   *Include Cumin in your meals. Cumin is great in chilli dishes, Indian and Chinese cuisine, on baked potatoes or roasted veg. You can use both whole Cumin seeds and ground Cumin.*

*Make a Cumin Tea by boiling one teaspoonful of Cumin seeds in 200 ml of water for 10 minutes. Let it cool and drink 2-3 cups a day.*

## Fennel

Fennel is widely used around the world. Fennel seeds act as laxative.

HOW TO USE ...   *Use both whole Fennel Seeds and ground Fennel in your kitchen for spicing your meals.*

*Chewing Fennel Seeds after your meal also help to*

*relieve constipation and bloating – chew one teaspoon of Fennel Seeds after dinner.*

### Fenugreek

Fenugreek is used both as an herb (the leaves) and as a spice (the seed). Fenugreek is native to South-eastern Europe and South Asia but today it grows in many parts of the world.

HOW TO USE ...

*Take two teaspoonfuls of fenugreek seeds powder with warm water in the morning and in the evening.*

*Sprinkle fresh Fenugreek leaves over your vegetable dishes and curries.*

*Include fresh Fenugreek leaves in your salads.*

*Sprout Fenugreek seeds and include them in your dishes.*

*Use Fenugreek leaves, both fresh and dried, in curries, dhal, vegetable dishes and chutneys.*

### Garlic

See page 43.

*Use fresh garlic in the kitchen. If fresh garlic is not available use ground garlic or garlic paste.*

### Ginger

Ginger spice has been used in Ayurvedic, herbal and traditional medicine for centuries as it has many medical qualities. Most of the Indian recipes and many of Chinese recipes use the ginger in one form or the other.

Both fresh and ground ginger is valuable to use in the kitchen. Fresh

HOW TO USE ... ginger is more recommended for stronger health properties.

Use Ginger in the salads, stir fries, curries, smoothies, juices etc.

## Tamarind

Tamarind is actually a fruit; it is also known as the **Indian Date** and grows primarily in India. We can usually find it in Asian markets in the form of whole pods, a compressed block, paste or concentrates. Tamarind has an extremely sour taste and can be used in the kitchen as the equivalent to lemon juice in preparing various dishes.

Tamarind is a powerful natural laxative.

HOW TO USE ... Tamarind can be eaten raw as it is considered as a fruit. Do not eat too many Tamarind pods as you may end up in the toilet with diarrhoea. In the store buy just closed Tamarind pods and make sure the pod color is closer to tan, not gray.

Use Tamarind in soups, bean dishes or chutneys.

Make your own Tamarind Juice - Place dry Tamarind into bowl, cover it with hot water and let it rest for 10 minutes. After soaking for 10 minutes start squeezing Tamarind with your hand for another 2 minutes. This way you will make Tamarind Juice which is great for relieving constipation. Strain and drink.

### Turmeric

Turmeric is known as a one of nature's most powerful healers and it is again one of the favourite spices commonly used in India.

HOW TO USE ...

*Use Turmeric in your kitchen for spicing your dishes.*

*Taking Turmeric with honey is also very effective – Mix half of teaspoon of Turmeric with one teaspoonful of honey and take it before meals.*

*Avoid Turmeric if you suffer by gallstones or bile obstruction. Avoid using Turmeric during pregnancy.*

### Whole Mustard Seeds

Mustard is also one of the oldest herbs used in traditional medicine. It was originally grown in China. In the 13th century Mustard appeared in Europe.

HOW TO USE ...

*Use Whole Mustard Seeds in your kitchen for spicing your meals.*

# Chapter 5: Recipes

 ## Folk Remedies

Here is a list of Folk Remedies which we inherited from our ancestors. The best way is to choose one or two remedy recipes and take them for one week or so. Soon you will see if they are the right remedies for you. Eventually you can change remedies one by one.

### Flax Seeds and Apple Cider Vinegar Mix
Place 1 tablespoonful of flaxseeds into boiling water and simmer until the substance will become jelly like. Once it cools down add 1 tablespoon of apple cider vinegar.
Drink in the morning.

### Flax seeds and oat bran Mix
Place 1 tablespoonful of flax seeds and 1 tablespoonful of oat bran into little bowl, cover the mixture with filtrated water and leave overnight. Eat this mixture in the morning half an hour before your breakfast. Do not forget to drink lots of water!

### Black Sesame Seeds with Honey
Grind black sesame seeds and mix them with honey. If you want you can make little balls from the mixture and eat them as sweets or take 1 tablespoon of the mixture 3 times a day.

### Sunflower Seeds Drink

Grind 2 tablespoonfuls of sunflower seeds and add them into the cup of boiling water. Add honey for better taste. Drink in the morning and before bedtime.

### Figs, Prunes and Dates Mixed in Liquorice Tea

Cut dried figs, dates and prunes into small cubes, place into the bowl and pour liquorice tea over it (you can buy liquorice tea bags in your health store or see page 63). Have this effective laxative snack twice a day in the morning and before bedtime.

### Prune Mix

For the Prune Mix you will need ½ cup of prunes, pitted and cut in small pieces, 1 teaspoonful of ground cinnamon, juice form ½ a lemon and 400 ml of filtrated water.

Bring water to boil, add prunes, ground cinnamon and simmer for 15 minutes. Stir in the lemon juice once it cools down.

Eat before bedtime.

### Dried Fruit Mix

*½ cup raisins*

*½ cup prunes, pitted.*

*½ cup dried dates, pitted*

*½ cup prune juice*

*¼ cup fresh orange juice (not from concentrate)*

Steam raisins, prunes and dried dates over boiling water to soften. Put into blender, add orange juice and prune juice and blend until smooth.

Eat this mixture on its own as a healthy snack, or spread over your oat crackers, or add into your morning porridge.

Can be refrigerated. Do not take this mixture for more than 10 days.

### Fruit Diet
Stay on the fruit diet for three to seven days. Eat all the fruits you like (except bananas and jack fruit), drink plenty of water and fruit juices.

 ## Herbs/ Teas to drink

Herbs and herbal teas listed below are the most effective ones for maintaining the digestive tract and for constipation relief.

You can stick to one or two herbal teas of your choice or you can combine them as much as you like. Drink at least three cups of herbal tea a day.
Teas mentioned here can be found in any decent health store or supermarkets pre-packed or in tea bags. If you buy the herbal tea bags, follow the preparation instruction from the label.
In the case you would buy just pure herbs, follow the preparation instruction stated below.

### Fresh Ginger Tea
Infuse 1 tablespoonful peeled and grated fresh root ginger in 200ml of boiling water for 10-15 minutes. Strain and drink three times a day.

### Dandelion Tea

Place 1/2 - 2 teaspoonfuls of dried or fresh grinded dandelion root into 200ml of boiling water for 10-15 minutes. Strain and drink three times a day.

### Barberry Tea

Infuse 2 teaspoonfuls of dried Barberry root or 2 teaspoonfuls of dried and crushed Barberry berries in 200ml of boiling water for 15 minutes. Strain before drinking. Drink two cups a day for no longer than 10 days.
Avoid using Barberry Tea during pregnancy.

### Burdock Tea

Place one teaspoonful of the Burdock root into a 200ml of water, bring to boil and simmer for 10-15 minutes. Strain and drink three times a day.

### Elderflower Tea

Infuse 2 teaspoonfuls of dried elderflower in 200ml of boiling water for 10-15 minutes. Strain before drinking. Take three times a day.

### Chickweed Tea

Infuse 1 tablespoon of dried or 3 tablespoons of fresh herb in 200ml boiling water and steep for 10 minutes. Strain and drink three times a day.

### Liquorice Tea

Infuse 1 teaspoonful of Liquorice root or powder in 200ml of boiling water for 10-15 minutes. Strain and drink 2-3 times a day before meals.

Liquorice is not recommended during pregnancy as it may increase the risk of premature delivery.

### Basil Tea

Infuse 2 teaspoonfuls of dried basil leafs or 8 fresh basil leafs in 200ml of boiling water for 10 minutes. Strain and drink three times a day.

Avoid using Basil Tea during Pregnancy.

### Flaxseeds/Linseed Tea

Place 3 tablespoons of flaxseeds/linseeds into a pot with 1 litre of water and bring to the boil. Turn of the heat and leave for at least 8 hours or overnight. After 8 hours bring it back to boil and simmer gently for 20 minutes. Once the tea cools down pass it through a sieve to remove the seeds.

Drink the tea throughout the day. It can be thinned with little bit of fresh water to make it easier to drink. You can also add little bit of honey and lemon juice for better taste.

Linseed Tea has a gelatinous consistence, strong taste and is an excellent colon lubricant. It aids overcoming constipation.

### Chamomile Tea

Infuse 2 teaspoonfuls of dried chamomile in 200ml of boiling water for 10-15 minutes. Strain before drinking. Take three times a day.

### Fennel Tea

Boil 2 teaspoonfuls of fennel seeds in 200ml of water for 20 minutes. Strain and drink three times a day.

### Peppermint Tea

Infuse 2 teaspoonfuls of dried peppermint in 200ml of boiling water for 10 minutes. Strain before drinking. Take three times a day.

### Nettle Tea

Fill the bigger cup or tea pot full of young nettle leaves, pour on boiling water and keep covered for 10 minutes. Strain and drink three times a day.

### Yellow Dock Tea

Boil 2 teaspoonfuls of Yellow Dock root for 10 minutes in 200ml of water. Strain and drink three times a day.

Yellow Dock Tea aids digestion and promotes bowel movements.

### Cardamom, Ginger and Cinnamon Tea

Put 10 pulverized cardamom seeds in 400ml of boiling water, add 2 teaspoons of fresh grinded ginger and one cinnamon stick. Simmer for 15 minutes. Sweeten with honey. Drink three cups a day.

### Constipation Mixture Tea

Mix together 2 parts of Dandelion root, 1 part of Yellow Dock root, 1 part of Burdock root, 1 part of Ginger root, and 1 part of Liquorice root.

Place 2 teaspoonfuls of the mixture in 200ml of boiling water and simmer for 5 minutes. Leave it covered for another 15 minutes. Strain and drink warm three times a day.

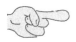

## Juices and Smoothies recipes

Juices and Smoothies are brilliant energy boosters full of vitamins, minerals and nutrients. They are also great for constipation relief.

## Juices

Have a glass of freshly made juice every morning and before bedtime. Feel free to make more juices for yourself during the day if possible.

**Carrot Juice** – Carrot Juice contains certain oils which have a beneficial effect on the mucous membranes in the stomach and intestines. This helps digestion and the bowels function properly.
Juice 3-4 carrots, makes 1 serving.

**Carrot and Celery Juice** – A great nutritional drink for relieving constipation is Carrot and Celery Juice. Celery helps to relax colon nerves and restore nerve function of the colon wall.
Juice 2-3 carrots and 1 celery stalk, makes 1 serving.

**Wheat Grass Juice** – Wheat Grass Juice is also great for relieving constipation. It is amazing energiser packed with vitamins and minerals and it is one of the best juices for the body detox.
Have a little "shot" of the Wheat Grass Juice every morning if possible.

**_Cabbage Juice_** – Cabbage Juice is anti-bacterial, helps to heal tissues in the stomach, intestines and colon and relieves constipation.

Juice ½ medium size cabbage, makes 1 serving. Add carrot, apple, basil or fennel for better flavour.

**_Lemon and Cayenne Pepper Drink_** – Lemon and Cayenne Pepper Drink improves the whole body health and wellbeing. It relieves constipation and stomach complains.

Mix a lemon juice from ½ a lemon, 250 ml filtrated water, 1/3 teaspoon ground Cayenne Pepper (you can use more if you have a strong stomach), and 1 teaspoon of honey if required. Have this drink first thing in the morning and before bedtime.

**_Boysenberry Juice_** – A boysenberry is a purple-blue berry a cross between raspberry and a Pacific blackberry. Boysenberry Juice has a mild laxative action. Include Boysenberry juice in your diet. You can buy it in your Health store or on internet.

**_Vitamin Booster_**

*7 carrots*
*5 tomatoes*
*3 celery stalks*
*2 garlic cloves*
*1 small onion*

Juice the carrots, tomatoes, celery, garlic and onion in the juice extractor. Makes 2 glasses.

**_Veggie Juice_**

*8 carrots*
*2 celery stalks*
*1 large cucumber*

1 cup parsley

1 small piece ginger

Juice all the ingredients together in the juice extractor and enjoy! Makes 2 glasses.

 ### Green Veggie Juice

6 celery stalks

1 cucumber

1 yellow pepper

½ cup baby spinach

½ cup cabbage

Juice the celery stalks, cucumber, yellow pepper, baby spinach and cabbage in the juice extractor and enjoy! Makes 2 glasses.

 ### Carrot, Orange and Cardamom Juice

4 oranges, peeled

7 carrots

pinch of ground cardamom

1 teaspoon honey

1 teaspoon natural vanilla extract

Juice the carrots and oranges in the juice extractor. Stir in the ground cardamom, honey and vanilla extract. Makes 2 glasses.

 ### Beetroot, Carrot and Ginger Juice

2 bigger beetroots

7 carrots,

3 cm piece ginger, peeled

Juice the beetroot, carrots and ginger. Makes 2 glasses.

 ### Spinach Mix Juice

2 cups baby spinach leaves

1 bigger or 2 smaller beetroots

8 carrots

2 celery stalks

2 apples

Juice all the ingredients together and enjoy! Makes 2 larger glasses.

 ### *Prune Drink*

150 g pitted prunes

400 ml water

2 teaspoons honey (optional)

1 teaspoon ground cinnamon

Blend prunes with water in the blender until smooth, add ground cinnamon and honey. Makes 2 larger glasses.

 ### *Spinach, Carrot and Apple Tango*

1 cup Spinach leaves

½ cup iceberg lettuce leafs

6 carrots

2 apples

2 celery stalks

Juice the spinach leaves, iceberg lettuce, carrots, apples and celery stalks in the juice extractor. Makes 2 glasses.

 ### *Citrus Booster*

1 lime

1 lemon

1 ripe grapefruit

5 oranges

2-3 tablespoons honey

Juice the lime, lemon, grapefruits and oranges in the citrus press. Add honey to taste. Makes 2 glasses.

### *Green Dream*

*2 cucumbers*

*2 limes, peeled*

*2 garlic gloves*

*½ cup coriander leafs*

*1 avocado, peeled, stone removed*

*1/3 teaspoon ground cumin*

Juice the cucumbers, limes, garlic and coriander leaves through juice extractor. Transfer to a blender, add avocado and ground cumin and blend until smooth. Makes 2 bigger glasses.

 ### *Health in the Glass*

*5 carrots*

*1 cucumber*

*2 apples*

*1 celery stalk*

*2 small beetroots, scrubbed*

Juice the carrots, cucumbers, apples, celery stalks and beetroots through a juice extractor. Makes 2 glasses.

## Smoothies

### *Berry Smoothie*

*10 strawberries*

*½ cup raspberries*

*½ cup blueberries*

*1 ripe pear*

*1 apple*

*1 tablespoon flax seeds*

*1 teaspoon sesame seeds*

*1 teaspoon (or more) Extra Virgin Olive Oil or Flaxseed Oil*

*200 ml water or apple juice (not from concentrate)*

Blend all the ingredients until smooth.

### **Pineapple and Mango Smoothie**

*1 cup fresh sliced pineapple*

*1 mango*

*½ cup berries (blueberries, raspberries, blackberries, etc.)*

*small piece fresh ginger*

*1 tablespoon oat bran*

*1 tablespoon flax seeds*

*1 teaspoon sunflower seeds*

*1 teaspoon Extra Virgin Olive Oil or Flaxseed Oil*

*300 ml pineapple or apple juice (not from concentrate)*

Blend all the ingredients until smooth.

### **Plum Smoothie**

*5 plums*

*2 nectarines*

*2 pears*

*1 tablespoon flax seeds*

*1 teaspoon sesame seeds*

*1 teaspoon Extra Virgin Olive Oil or Flaxseed Oil*

*200 ml water or fruit juice (not from concentrate)*

Blend all the ingredients until smooth.

### *Peach and Mango Smoothie*

*1 mango*

*3 peaches*

*½ cup blueberries*

*1 tablespoon flaxseeds*

*1 teaspoon Extra Virgin Olive Oil or Flaxseed Oil*

*250 ml water or peach juice (not from concentrate)*

Blend all the ingredients until smooth.

 ### *Peach and Apricot Smoothie*

*2 peaches*

*7 fresh apricots or 1 cup dried apricots (soak dried apricots in the water overnight)*

*1 tablespoon flaxseeds*

*1 teaspoon sunflower seeds*

*1 teaspoon Extra Virgin Olive Oil or Flaxseed Oil*

*300 ml water or peach juice (not from concentrate)*

Blend all the ingredients until smooth.

 ### *Coconut and Pineapple Smoothie*

*½ cup coconut meat*

*1 cup pineapple*

*1 teaspoon ground cinnamon*

*1 teaspoon oat bran*

*1 tablespoon flaxseeds*

*1 teaspoon Extra Virgin Olive Oil or Flaxseed Oil*

*250 ml water or pineapple or apple juice (not from concentrate)*

Blend all the ingredients until smooth.

### Kale Smoothie

1 cup Kale

½ cup green grapes

2 pears

1 orange

10 mint leaves

1 tablespoon flax seeds

1 teaspoon sesame seeds

1 teaspoon sunflower seeds

1 teaspoon Extra Virgin Olive Oil or Flaxseed Oil

250 ml water


Blend all the ingredients until smooth.

### Apple-Spinach Smoothie

2 green apples

1 cup baby spinach

2 pears

½ banana

1 tablespoon flaxseeds

1 tablespoon oat bran

1 teaspoon Extra Virgin Olive Oil or Flaxseed Oil

200 ml walnut or rice milk


Blend all the ingredients until smooth.

### Cucumber and Kale Smoothie

½ cucumber

1 cup kale or baby spinach

2 green apples

½ cup green grapes

1 tablespoon flax seeds

*1 teaspoon sesame seeds*

*1 teaspoon sunflower seeds*

*1 teaspoon Extra Virgin Olive Oil or Flaxseed Oil*

*200 ml apple juice (not from concentrate)*

Blend all the ingredients until smooth.

 ## Green Smoothie

*1 bunch dandelion greens*

*½ cucumber*

*1 lime or lemon*

*2 green apples*

*1 tablespoon flax seeds*

*1 tablespoon oat bran*

*1 teaspoon sunflower seeds*

*1 teaspoon Extra Virgin Olive Oil or Flaxseed Oil*

*250 ml apple juice (not from concentrate)*

Blend all the ingredients until smooth.

 ## Rice Milk Smoothie

*3 peaches*

*1 mango*

*1 tablespoon flax seeds*

*1 teaspoon sunflower seeds*

*1 teaspoon oat bran*

*1 teaspoon Extra Virgin Olive Oil or Flaxseed Oil*

*300 ml Rice Milk*

Blend all the ingredients until smooth.

**_Salads recipes_**

Salads are an important part of our diet. They contain dietary fibre, vitamins, minerals, nutrients and **_life enzymes_** which are not destroyed by cooking process.

Salad is the one of the best foods for a healthy body. Salad dressings should be made from some type of cold pressed oil.

If you are thinking about changing your diet to more healthy one full of vegetables and fruits you will need to eat bigger portions as vegetables and fruits have less calories then chips and steak or pizza. It is better to have a big bowl of salad and feel satisfied then just a small one and after a short while crave for crisps or chocolate bar.

You can use plenty of vegetable variations in your Salads.

For constipation relief it is best to use green leafy vegetables such as spinach, kale or cabbage, then celery, beetroot, carrots, tomatoes, red onions, or courgettes (zucchinis).

### _Spinach and Strawberry Salad_

_4 cups baby spinach leafs_

_2 cups strawberries, sliced_

_25 g pecan halves, lightly toasted (optional)_

_25 g diced almonds_

_100 g goat cheese, cut in small dices (optional)_

_Dressing_

_½ cup Extra Virgin Olive Oil_

_4 tablespoons balsamic vinegar_

_3 tablespoon honey_

*1 teaspoon of dried tarragon*

*1 teaspoon of garlic powder*

Combine strawberries with spinach, pecan halves, almonds and goat cheese in a bowl. Blend Olive oil, balsamic vinegar, honey, tarragon and garlic powder in the blender and drizzle over the salad. Enjoy! Serves 2.

### Simple Spinach Salad

*3 cups baby spinach*

*1 cups kale*

*25 g pine nuts*

*25 g almonds*

*1/3 cup raisins or dried cranberries, diced dates or figs*

<u>*Dressing*</u>

*4 tablespoons Extra Virgin Olive Oil*

*4 tablespoon balsamic vinegar*

*1 teaspoon cider apple vinegar*

*4 tablespoons apple juice (not from concentrate)*

*1 tablespoon maple syrup (optional)*

*1 teaspoon fresh ground black pepper*

Soak raisins, cranberries, dates or figs in hot water for 15 minutes, drain. Toast pine nuts and almonds in a dry pan constantly stirring. Mix dressing ingredients together. In the large bowl mix baby spinach with kale, sprinkle over soaked raisins, cranberries, dates or figs, toasted pine nuts and almonds. Pour over the freshly made dressing and serve. Serves 2.

### Spinach and Avocado Salad

*4 cups baby spinach leafs*

*2 avocados, sliced*

*1 red onion, sliced*

*50 g walnuts*

<u>Dressing</u>

*¼ cup Extra Virgin Olive Oil or other cold pressed Oil*

*¼ cup fresh squeezed lemon juice*

*1 teaspoon apple cider vinegar*

*3 tablespoon fresh cut coriander*

Mix the baby spinach, avocados, red onion and walnuts in a big bowl. Whisk Extra Virgin Olive Oil, lemon juice, apple cider vinegar and coriander together and pour over the salad. Serves 2.

### Simple Cabbage Salad

*1 small head red cabbage*

*1 small head green cabbage*

<u>Dressing</u>

*Juice of 3 limes*

*1/3 cup Extra Virgin Olive Oil*

*Tamari or other type of soy sauce to taste*

*1/3 cup sesame seeds*

Slice the cabbages into thin strips. Whisk lime juice, olive oil, Tamari and sesame seeds together and toss with cabbage. Let it sit covered for at least 1 hour. Serves 2.

### Cabbage, Carrot and Raisins Salad

½ small head red or green cabbage

3 carrots

½ cucumbers

1 small Romaine lettuce

1/3 cup raisins

2 tablespoonfuls ground flax seeds

*Dressing*

1/2 cup Extra Virgin Olive Oil or another cold pressed Oil

4 tablespoons balsamic vinegar

1 tablespoon apple cider vinegar

Slice cabbage into thin strips, grate carrots, chop cucumber, and tear Romaine lettuce into small pieces, put all into a bowl. Add raisins and flax seeds. Whisk Extra Virgin Olive Oil, balsamic vinegar and apple cider vinegar together, pour over the salad and toss well. Let it sit for half an hour. Serves 2-3.

### Avocado Salad

2 avocados, sliced

2 cups baby spinach leafs

1 cup of other salad greens or lettuce or herbs

8 cherry tomatoes, sliced in half

½ carrots, shredded

50 g almonds, crushed

*Dressing*

1 avocado

1 vine tomato

1 small red onion

1 garlic clove

*2 tablespoons flax seeds*
*1/3 cup Extra Virgin Olive Oil or another cold pressed Oil*
*juice of 1 lime or 1 lemon*

Slice the avocados and mix them with spinach, greens, cherry tomatoes, and carrots in a big bowl.

Blend 1 avocado, vine tomato, red onion, garlic, flax seeds, lime or lemon juice and olive oil in blender and pour over the salad. Sprinkle with the crushed almonds. Serves 2.

### Simple Beetroot Salad
*500g pre-cooked beetroot.*

*Dressing*
*5 tablespoons Extra Virgin Olive Oil*
*2 tablespoons apple cider vinegar*
*1 teaspoon cumin seeds*
*Pinch ground black pepper*
Slice the beetroot into thin strips, put into a bowl. Add Extra Virgin Olive Oil, apple cider vinegar, cumin seeds and ground black pepper. Toss well and let it sit for half an hour. Serves 2.

### Beetroot and Apples
*3 fresh beetroots*
*4 apples*
*2 tablespoons pumpkin seeds*
*2 tablespoon flaxseeds*

*Dressing*
*¼ cup Extra Virgin Olive Oil or another cold pressed oil*
*Juice from 1 lime or lemon*
*1 teaspoon honey*

Peel the beetroots and apples and grate them on the grater. Place them into the bowl. Add pumpkin seeds and flaxseeds.

Whisk Extra Virgin Olive Oil with lime juice and honey. Pour the mixture over the beetroots and apples and toss well.

### *Romaine Lettuce with Chickpea*

*1 small Romaine lettuce (or Iceberg lettuce)*

<u>*Dressing*</u>

*4 garlic cloves*

*4 tablespoons cooked chickpea (can be from tin)*

*1 tablespoon capers*

*2 tablespoons flaxseeds*

*¼ cup Extra Virgin Olive Oil*

*2 teaspoons Tamari*

*Juice from 1 lime or lemon*

*Pinch ground black pepper*

*Fried Polenta croutons*

Blend the garlic, chickpea, capers, flaxseeds, Extra Virgin Olive Oil, Tamari and lime juice in the blender. Tear the Romaine lettuce and put into a bowl. Pour over the mixture from the blender and toss well. Garnish with ground black pepper and Polenta croutons. Serves 2.

### *Dinner Salad*

*1 cup cooked lentils*

*2 cups baby spinach*

*4 small pre-cooked beetroots*

*3 carrots*

*1 red onion*

*4 garlic cloves*

<u>Dressing</u>
*1/3 cup Extra Virgin Olive Oil*
*2 tablespoons red wine vinegar*
*1 tablespoon apple cider vinegar*
*2 tablespoons flaxseeds*
*Fresh herbs – basil, thyme, or rosemary*

Place cooked lentils and baby spinach into a big bowl. Cut beetroots into thin slices, grate carrots, dice onion and garlic and add into the bowl. Whisk Extra Virgin Olive Oil with wine vinegar, apple cider vinegar, flaxseeds and herbs and pour over the salad. Toss well. Serves 2.

## *Tuna Salad*

*200 g tin tuna steak*
*2 cups baby spinach leaves*
*1 cup watercress leaves*
*1 cup rocket leaves*
*½ cucumber*
*10 cherries tomatoes*
*3 tablespoons fresh dill*
*2 tablespoons sunflower seeds*

<u>Dressing</u>
*Juice of ½ lemon*
*1/3 cup Extra Virgin Olive Oil*

Mix the leaves in the big bowl. Add the drained Tuna, halved cherry tomatoes, sliced cucumber, chopped dill and sunflower seeds. Toss well. Drizzle with lemon juice and Extra Virgin Olive Oil. Serves 2.

 ## Breakfast, Lunch or Snack Fruit Salads

### Berries and Apple Salad
6 apples, cored
2 peaches
1 cup of berries (blueberries, raspberries, strawberries, etc.)
2 teaspoonful ground cinnamon
Pinch of nutmeg
¼ cup nuts (it can be walnuts, almonds, macadamias, pistachios, Brazil nuts, hazelnuts, cashews, or pecans)
300 ml non-dairy probiotic yogurt
Add a few mint leafs to garnish

Cut up the apples and peaches and put them into a bowl. Add berries, nuts, spices, and yogurt. Mix together and garnish with mint leafs. Serves 2-3.

### Green Fruit Salad
4 apples
Big bunch of green grapes
2 stalks of celery
1 spring of fresh mint
1/3 cup pistachios, shelled
2 tablespoons fresh lemon juice
1 tablespoon honey or maple syrup, optional

Cut all the grapes in half and put into a big bowl. Cut the celery stalks and apples into little bite-sized pieces, cut mint leafs into thin strips and add them all into the bowl with grapes. Add pistachios, lemon juice, maple syrup or honey and mix well.
Serves 2.

## *Mix Fruit Salad*

*1/4 pineapple*
*1 grapefruit*
*1 mango*
*1 apple*
*2 kiwis*
*2 peaches*
*1 orange*
*1 lime or 1 lemon*
*2 tablespoons fresh ginger, minced*
*2 tablespoons fresh mint, minced*
*1/3 cup sesame seeds*

Cut all the fruits into little bite-sized pieces and put into a bowl. Whisk lime juice with ginger, mint and sesame seeds and pour over the fruits. Toss well and let it sit for 15 minutes. Serves 2.

## *Lunch Fruit Salad*

*1 small Romaine lettuce*
*4 peaches*
*big bunch of red grapes*
*1/3 pineapple*
*1 sliced bananas, optional*
*1/4 cup of walnuts*
*1/4 cup of pecans*
*1/4 cup of sunflower seeds*

*1/3 cup of shredded coconut*

Tear the Romaine lettuce, cut peaches, pineapple and bananas into little bite-sized pieces, cut all grapes in half and mix all in a big bowl. Add walnuts, pecans, sunflower seeds and shredded coconut. Serves 2-3.

### Persimmon Lunch Salad

| | |
|---|---|
| *4 persimmons* | *¼ cup cranberries or raisins* |
| *1 mango* | *¼ cup crushed almonds* |
| *2 apples* | *3 tablespoonfuls oat bran* |
| *1 pear* | *½ bag Mix-Leafs Salad* |
| *seeds from 1 pomegranate* | *1 lime or lemon* |
| *1 avocado* | |

Cut all the fruit and avocado into bite size pieces and put into a bowl. Add a mix of leafs, cranberries, pomegranate seeds, and oat bran and toss well. Pour the lime or lemon juice over the salad and sprinkle with crushed almonds. Serves 2-3.

### Breakfast Fruit Salad

| | |
|---|---|
| *2 red apples* | *15 almonds, crushed* |
| *2 green apples* | *3 tablespoons ground flaxseeds* |
| *1 pear* | *3 tablespoons of Goji berries* |
| *bunch of grapes* | *1 orange* |
| *¼ cup raisins* | *1 lime* |

Cut apples and pear into bite size pieces, cut all grapes in half, and place into a bowl. Add raisins, almonds and flax seeds and toss well. Squeeze the orange and the lime over the salad. Serves 2.

### Simple Breakfast/Snack Mix

*1 mango*
*3 kiwis*
*10 strawberries*
*2 tablespoons ground flaxseeds*
*3 tablespoons shredded dried coconut*
*2 tablespoons oat bran flakes*
*Maple syrup*

Cut mango, kiwis and strawberries into bite size pieces, and place into a bowl. Add flaxseeds, coconut, oat bran and Maple syrup and toss well. Serves 1-2.

### Quick Apple Snack

*3 apples*
*2 tablespoons raisins*
*2 tablespoons ground cinnamon*
*Juice from half a lemon*

Peel and grate the apples, put into a bowl. Add raisins, ground cinnamon, lemon juice and toss well. Serves 1.

### Carrot-Fruit Salad

*3 carrots*
*4 apples*
*¼ pineapple*
*1 orange*

*10 dates*
*2 tablespoons sunflower seeds*
*2 tablespoons flaxseeds*
*Juice from 1 lime or lemon*

Grate the carrots, apples, and place them into a bowl. Cut the pineapple, orange and dates into small bite size pieces and add into the bowl. Sprinkle with sunflower seeds and flaxseeds, pour over the lime or lemon juice and toss well. Serves 2-3.

### Fruit Heaven

| | |
|---|---|
| 3 peaches | Bunch green grapes |
| 20 strawberries | Juice of one lime |
| 1/3 pineapple | ½ cup pineapple juice |
| Bunch red grapes | 1 teaspoon ground ginger |

Cut the peaches, pineapple and strawberries into bite size pieces. Cut all grapes in half, place all into a bowel. Mix lime juice, pineapple juice and ground ginger together and pour over the fruits. Toss well. Serves 2-3.

### Stewed Prunes and Apples

200 g prunes, pitted
5 apples
2 teaspoons ground cinnamon
2 teaspoons honey, optional
¾ cup filtrated water
Juice of half a lemon

In the saucepan, combine the prunes, sliced apples, honey, and water. Cook over medium heat until the prunes are plump and apples soft. Transfer prunes and apples into two serving bowls, drizzle with the lemon juice and sprinkle with the ground cinnamon. Serves 2.

**Soups recipes**

Vegetable soups are great source of soluble fibre and provide additional liquid moistening for the intestines. Soups help to maintain the alkaline ph and restore the bowel balance. Some vegetable soups have a mild laxative effect.

### Spinach Soup

*300g spinach, can be fresh or frozen*

*2 onions*

*4 potatoes*

*500 ml vegetable stock*

*1 teaspoon ground nutmeg*

*½ teaspoon ground black pepper*

*Little bit coconut oil*

*Extra Virgin Olive Oil to drizzle, to taste*

Peel and chop the potatoes and boil until soft. Peel and chop the onion and fry in saucepan on coconut oil until see through. Add spinach into saucepan, fry for one more minute, and then add vegetable stock, nutmeg, and ground pepper. Boil until spinach is wilted. Add potatoes. Use hand blender and blend the soup until smooth. Once is served drizzle over with Extra Virgin Olive Oil.

### Red Lentil Soup

*350g split red lentils*

*3 pints vegetable stock*

*1 large onion*

*2 garlic cloves*

*2 carrots*

*1 teaspoon ground cumin*

*1 teaspoon ground coriander*

*½ teaspoon cayenne pepper*

*½ teaspoon black pepper*

*Juice from ½ lemon*

*Extra Virgin Olive Oil to drizzle, to taste*

Put the lentils, chopped onion, garlic gloves, chopped carrots, and vegetable stock into a big saucepan and boil for half an hour. Add seasoning and more water if soup needs thinning. Boil for another 3 minutes. Add lemon juice. Use hand blender to blend the soup until smooth. Once served, drizzle over with Extra Virgin Olive Oil.

### Pumpkin and Onion Soup

*1 medium pumpkin or large butternut squash*
*1 large onion*
*500 ml vegetable stock*
*½ teaspoon cayenne pepper, optional*
*½ teaspoon black pepper*
*1 tablespoon coconut oil*
*Extra Virgin Olive Oil to drizzle, to taste*

Chop the onion finely. Peel and de-seed the pumpkin or butternut squash and chop into chunks. Heat the coconut oil in the saucepan and fry the onion until see through. Add the pumpkin or squash and cook for a further five minutes. Add vegetable stock and seasoning, and simmer until the pumpkin is soft. Add more water if soup needs thinning. Use hand blender to blend the soup until smooth. Once served, drizzle over with Extra Virgin Olive Oil.

### Sweet Pea Soup

*350g fresh or frozen peas*
*1 carrot*
*1 potato*
*2 onions*
*2 garlic cloves*
*1 small tin (125ml) sweet corn niblets*
*¾ litre vegetable stock*

*3 tablespoon fresh tarragon*

*½ teaspoon cayenne pepper, optional*

*½ teaspoon black pepper*

*1 tablespoon coconut oil*

*Extra Virgin Olive Oil to drizzle, to taste*


Chop the onion and garlic cloves finely, dice carrot and potato. Heat the coconut oil in the large saucepan and sauté the onion, garlic and carrot until softened. Add potato, peas, seasoning and vegetable stock and simmer for 20 minutes. Add more water if soup needs thinning. Add sweet corn niblets and simmer for another 5 minutes. Use hand blender to blend the soup until smooth. Once served, drizzle over with Extra Virgin Olive Oil.

### Vegetable and lentil Soup

| | |
|---|---|
| *2 leeks* | *3 vine tomatoes* |
| *2 carrots* | *200g whole brown or green lentils* |
| *1 parsnip* | *1 litre vegetable stock* |
| *4 celery stalks* | *1 tablespoon fresh thyme* |
| *1 small sweet potato* | *1 tablespoon fresh marjoram* |
| *1 onion* | *½ teaspoon black pepper* |
| *3 garlic cloves* | |
| *1 tin of chopped tomatoes* | |
| *2 tablespoons coconut oil* | |


Chop the leeks, carrots, parsnip, celery stalks, sweet potato and vine tomatoes into small pieces. Chop the onion finely and crush garlic cloves. Heat the coconut oil in the large saucepan and sauté the onion, garlic and leeks for 5 minutes. Add vegetable stock, carrots, parsnip, celery stalks, sweet potato, tomatoes, lentils and black pepper and simmer for 15 minutes. Add more water if soup needs thinning. Add marjoram and thyme and simmer for another 10 minutes. Serve.

### Carrot and Coriander Soup

*10 medium carrots*
*1 large onion*
*Bunch of fresh coriander*
*½ teaspoon cayenne pepper, optional*
*½ teaspoon black pepper*
*1 litre vegetable stock*
*1 tablespoon coconut oil*
*Extra Virgin Olive Oil to drizzle, to taste*
*Sesame seeds to garnish*

Heat the coconut oil in a big saucepan, chop onion finely and fry until see through. Peel and chop the carrots and add them into a saucepan. Add vegetable stock, seasoning and simmer for 20 minutes. Add more water if soup needs thinning. Add coriander and simmer for another 3 minutes. Use hand blender to blend the soup until smooth. Once served, drizzle over with Extra Virgin Olive Oil and sprinkle with sesame seeds.

### Vegetable and Butter Bean Soup

*1 tin butter beans*
*1 carrot*
*1 medium potato*
*200 g cabbage*
*1 onion*
*3 tablespoons pesto*
*½ teaspoon turmeric*
*½ teaspoon curry powder*
*½ teaspoon ground black pepper*

1 teaspoon Worcestershire sauce
Vegetable stock


Chop the carrot, potato, cabbage and onion and put them into a big saucepan. Cover with vegetable stock, add seasoning and simmer for 20 minutes. Use hand blender to blend the soup until smooth and serve.

### Bean and Vegetable Soup

400 g can borlotti beans or other type of beans
400 g fresh spinach
1 tin chopped tomatoes
1 courgette
2 celery sticks
1 fennel bulb
2 carrots
2 onions
5 garlic cloves
3 tablespoons coconut oil
½ teaspoon black ground pepper
1 litre vegetable stock


Chop the courgette, celery sticks, fennel, carrots, and onions and crush the garlic cloves. Heat coconut oil in a big saucepan, add onions, carrots, celery, fennel and garlic and fry for 5 minutes. Add the courgette and fry for another 2 minutes. Stir in the beans, tomatoes, pesto and vegetable stock and simmer for half an hour. Add more water if soup needs thinning.
Stir-fry the spinach separately in the frying pan for 1-2 minutes. Place it into the soup bowls, ladle the soup over the spinach and sprinkle with ground black pepper and serve.

### Tomato Basil Bean Soup

10 vine tomatoes

1 tin kidney beans or other type of beans

1 onion

3 garlic cloves

½ cup fresh basil

½ cup fresh baby spinach

2 bay leafs

½ litre vegetable stock

½ teaspoon ground black pepper

1 tablespoon coconut oil

Extra Virgin Olive Oil to drizzle, to taste

Chop tomatoes and onion, crush garlic. Heat coconut oil in a saucepan and fry onion until see through. Add garlic, tomatoes, beans, vegetable stock and bay leafs and simmer for 15 minutes. Add more water if soup needs thinning. Add basil and spinach and simmer until they wilt. Once served; drizzle over with Extra Virgin Olive Oil and sprinkle with ground black pepper.

### Sauerkraut Soup

500 g sauerkraut

2 leaves of Savoy cabbage

1 celery stalk

1 carrot

1 small leek

10 button mushrooms

6 shiitake mushrooms

10 tomatoes

1 litre water

3 bay leafs

1/2 teaspoon caraway seed

*3 tablespoons Extra Virgin Olive Oil*

If your sauerkraut is too sour, rinse it first, and then put into a big saucepan. Cut all the rest vegetables into bite size pieces and put them all into the saucepan. Add seasoning and cover with water. Simmer for an hour. Eventually add a little more water if needed. Drizzle Extra Virgin Olive Oil over the soup and serve.

### Carrot Ginger Soup

*6 carrots*
*3 cm piece ginger*
*1 parsnip*
*1 celery stalk*
*1 onion*
*3 garlic cloves*
*2 bay leafs*
*1 teaspoon ground coriander*
*½ teaspoon black pepper*
*700 ml (or more) vegetable stock*
*Extra Virgin Olive Oil to drizzle, to taste*

Peel and cut the carrots and parsnip. Peel and mince the ginger. Cut celery stalk and onion into smaller pieces.

Put all the vegetables into a big saucepan, add seasoning and cover with vegetable stock. Simmer for half an hour. Take out the bay leafs and blend the soup until smooth with the hand blender. Drizzle Extra Virgin Olive Oil over the soup and serve.

**Dinner Tips**

If you suffer from constipation your dinner should be light, not highly processed, or deep fried. Your dinner should not contain white flour, red meat, or mucous forming foods such as dairy products. Starchy foods should be also avoided.

Feel free to have salads or vegetable soups for your dinner anytime you like.
Here are some healthy dinner recipe tips.

### Butter Bean, Tomato and Olive Stew

1 ½ tin butter beans

1 punnet cherry tomatoes

½ cup black olives, pitted

2 small onions

4 garlic cloves

1 small piece ginger

3 tablespoons coconut oil

1 teaspoon honey

½ teaspoon fresh black pepper

Pinch of saffron threads

1 teaspoon sweet paprika

1 teaspoon ground cinnamon

1 teaspoon sesame seeds

Fresh flat leaf parsley to garnish

Heat the coconut oil in the saucepan. Add finely chopped onion, ginger and crushed garlic, and cook for 5-10 minutes until softened. Stir in whole cherry tomatoes, rinsed and dried butter beans, saffron threads, sweet paprika, ground cinnamon, black pepper and honey. Cook until tomatoes are soft. Stir in black olives and cook for another 1-2 minutes. Sprinkle with sesame seeds and garnish with fresh parsley. Serves 2.

### Salmon Steak covered in Mango Salsa

*2 salmon steaks*
*1 mango*
*2 spring onions or 2 small red onions*
*½ cucumber*
*3 tablespoons fresh chopped coriander*
*½ teaspoon black pepper*
*juice of 1 lime*
*2 lemon wedges and fresh coriander to garnish*

Mango Salsa

Chop the mango flesh into small cubes. Finely chop cucumber, spring or red onions, and parsley. Place them all into a bowl, sprinkle with black pepper and toss. Cover and let it rest for half an hour.

Place the Salmon Steak on the grill pan, drizzle over the lime juice and cook for about 5-6 minutes on each side until tender.
Once served, cover Salmon Steaks with Mango Salsa, garnish with fresh parsley and lemon wedges.
Serve with fresh vegetable salad or steamed vegetables such as asparagus, sweet peas, carrots, etc.
Serves 2.

### Chinese Cabbage Casserole

*500 g Chinese cabbage*
*100 g daikon or radish*

*3 carrots*

*2 garlic cloves*

*2 cm piece ginger*

*30 g arame seaweed*

*1 bunch fresh coriander*

*1 teaspoon coriander seeds*

*1 teaspoon sesame seeds*

*1 teaspoon sesame oil*

*1 teaspoon soy-sauce (wheat free)*

*1 litre water*

Soak arame seaweed overnight in the water.

Tear Chinese cabbage and put into a big saucepan. Add sliced carrots, sliced daikon, sliced ginger, coriander seeds, garlic, and cover it with water. Bring it to boil and simmer for 10-15 minutes. Lastly, stir in fresh coriander. Once is served drizzle over the sesame oil, soy sauce, sesame seeds and arame. Serves 2.

### Herb Baked Cod

*2 bigger cod fillets*

*2 big vine tomatoes*

*½ teaspoon black pepper*

*mix of dried herbs – oregano, thyme, basil, coriander, marjoram, dill, mint, etc.*

*juice of ½ lemon*

Place the cod fillets into a small baking tray. Cover them with mixed herbs, season with black pepper, and top with sliced tomatoes. Cover with the foil. Bake in the 200°C preheated oven for 15-20 minutes until the fish is cooked. Once is served drizzle over the lemon juice.

Serve with the salads or steamed or roasted vegetables. Serves 2.

96

### Chayote and Courgette (Zucchini) Stir-Fry

1 chayote

1 courgette

1 butter squash or 2 small crookneck squashes

1 onion

1 tablespoon sesame seeds

1 teaspoon dried oregano or 3 tablespoon fresh oregano

1 teaspoon dried basil or 3 tablespoons fresh basil

½ teaspoon fresh black pepper

2 tablespoons coconut oil

Extra Virgin Olive Oil to drizzle, to taste


Heat coconut oil in a big frying pan. Chop onion, add into the frying pan and fry for 2 minutes. Chop chayote, add into the pan and fry for another 2 minutes. Chop the courgette and butter or crookneck squash, add into the frying pan. Stir in seasoning, cover and cook for 12-15 minutes until the vegetables are soft. Once is served sprinkle with sesame seeds and drizzle with Extra Virgin Olive Oil. Serves 2.


### Veggie Casserole

150 g cauliflower florets

1 small courgette

1 tin red kidney beans

1 tin chick peas

1 tin chopped tomatoes

1 green pepper

1 large onion

4 garlic cloves

1 teaspoon ground cumin

1 teaspoon dried thyme

1 teaspoon dried oregano

½ teaspoon black pepper

½ teaspoon cayenne pepper

1 teaspoon honey

2 tablespoons flaxseeds or sesame seeds

Extra Virgin Olive Oil to drizzle, to taste


Chop the onion, green pepper and courgette, mince the garlic, and drain the beans and chick peas. Combine all the ingredients in the large casserole dish and bake in the 200°C preheated oven for 45 minutes until all vegetables are soft.

You may add diced goats cheese on the top of casserole if you like the last 10 minutes of baking. Once served, drizzle over with Extra Virgin Olive Oil to taste. Serves 3.

### Garlic – Ginger Buckwheat Noodles

1 pack buckwheat noodles

3 cups baby spinach

½ cup sugar peas

½ cup bean sprouts

3 cm piece fresh ginger

6 garlic cloves

1 small onion

4 tablespoons soy sauce

3 tablespoons Hoisin sauce (you will find it in Chinese shop)

2 tablespoons flaxseeds or sesame seeds

½ teaspoon black pepper

2-3 tablespoons coconut oil

Extra Virgin Olive Oil to drizzle, to taste

Few fresh mint leaves to garnish


Cook buckwheat noodles and set aside.

Chop the onion and ginger finely and crush the garlic cloves. Heat coconut oil in a big frying pan, add onion, garlic and ginger and stir fry for 2 minutes. Add the rest of vegetables, soy sauce, Hoisin sauce, flaxseeds or sesame seeds and black pepper and stir fry for another 5-8 minutes until all the vegetables are soft. Stir buckwheat noodles in last. Once is serve drizzle with Extra Virgin Olive Oil and garnish with mint leaves. Serves 2.

### Veggie Stir Fry

150 g broccoli florets
150 g cauliflower florets
10 baby carrots
1 red pepper
1 yellow pepper
10 mushrooms
1 bigger onion
4 garlic cloves
2 cm piece fresh ginger
Extra Virgin Olive Oil to drizzle, to taste

1 tablespoon lemon juice
2 tablespoons orange juice
1 tablespoon rice vinegar
2 tablespoons soy sauce
Little bit of water if needed
1-2 teaspoons honey
2 tablespoons sesame seeds
2 tablespoons coconut oil

Slice the baby carrots, peppers and mushrooms, chop onion, crush garlic cloves and mince the ginger.

Heat the coconut oil in a big saucepan or wok, add onion, garlic and ginger and stir fry for 2 minutes. Add rest of the vegetables, sesame seeds, lemon and orange juice, rice vinegar, soy sauce and the honey and stir fry for 10 minutes until all the vegetables are soft. Add little bit of water if needed. Once is served drizzle with Extra Virgin Olive Oil.

Serve on its own or with a little bowl of brown rice. Serves 2.

### Backed Fish Fillet

*750g fish fillet*
*7 fresh tomatoes or 1 ½ tins of chopped tomatoes*
*2 onions*
*4 cloves garlic*
*½ cup chopped parsley*
*10 fresh basil leafs or 2 teaspoons dried basil*
*1 teaspoon dried oregano*
*½ teaspoon black pepper*
*1 teaspoon honey*
*½ cup dry white wine*
*2-3 tablespoons coconut oil*

Peel and chop tomatoes, chop onions and mince the garlic. Heat the coconut oil in the frying pan, add onions, garlic and stir fry for 2 minutes. Add parsley, basil, oregano, black pepper, honey, white wine and tomatoes. Stir fry for another 5 minutes.

Arrange the fish fillets in the baking dish, cover with tomatoes mix and bake in preheated oven for 20-30 minutes until fish is cooked. Serve with fresh vegetable salad or steamed vegetables. Serves 2.

### Backed Herbed Sea Bass

*2 bigger sea bass fish with the head and tail left on*
*2 onions*
*3 garlic cloves*
*1 teaspoon dried marjoram leafs*
*1 teaspoon dried thyme leafs*
*1 teaspoon white pepper*
*4 bay leaves*
*½ cup of white wine*
*¼ cup coconut oil*
*Lime or lemon wedges to garnish*

100

Wash the fish and place into a backing dish. Chop onions, mince garlic and put them into a bowl. Add all the herbs, white wine, coconut oil and mix well. Pour the mixture over and inside the fish. Bake in 200°C preheated oven for 20-30 minutes until fish is cooked. Serve with fresh vegetable salad or steamed vegetables. Serves 2.

### Aubergine and Chick Pea Curry

1 tin chick peas

1 large aubergine

1 tin chopped tomatoes

1 large onion

3 garlic cloves

2 cm piece fresh ginger

2 fresh chillies

50g tomato puree

2 tablespoons coconut oil

1 teaspoon brown mustard seeds

1 teaspoon cumin seeds

1 teaspoon ground cumin

1 teaspoons ground coriander

1 teaspoons ground turmeric

½ teaspoon ground fenugreek

½ teaspoon cayenne pepper

1 bunch fresh coriander

Chop the onion, chillies, and aubergine, crush the garlic, mince the ginger and drain the chick peas. Heat coconut oil in a big saucepan, add cumin and mustard seeds and fry them until they are popping, add onion, stir well and fry for another 2 minutes. Blend garlic, chillies and ginger in the blender until smooth paste and add into saucepan. Cook for another 3 minutes. Add the rest of ingredients into the saucepan except fresh coriander, cover and simmer for another 30 minutes. Stir fresh chopped coriander in last and serve immediately. Serves 2.

# Chapter 6: Exercise

Physical activity is essential for our body health and wellbeing. Exercise gets the whole body moving including the inner organs and intestines. Exercise stimulates the peristalsis of the colon wall and helps the faecal matter move the right direction - out of the body.

- Exercise stimulates the release of epinephrine, a hormone that creates a sense of happiness and excitement thus, one becomes more relaxed and happier.
- Exercise helps with mood swings, reduces feelings of depression and anxiety.
- Exercise speeds up metabolism. Once a person exercises, he/she burns calories which lead to weight loss and a toned body.
- Exercise improves sleep by producing a significant rise in body temperature followed by a compensatory drop a few hours later. The drop in body temperature, which persists for two to four hours after exercise, makes it easier to fall asleep and stay asleep.
- Exercise strengthens and stimulates the heart and lungs, vitalizes the nervous system, sharpens the brain by increasing the amount of oxygen available, activates the endocrine system (helps lymph to move in lymphatic vessels), helps with toxin removal, can help to manage high blood pressure, prevent diabetes and osteoporosis.
- Exercise brings the better sex life by boosting the energy and strengthening the pelvic muscles.

*Your body should be exercised every day ideally.*

*The best is to find a type of exercise you like as exercises should be pleasure and fun.*

*Before you begin a new form of exercise consult your doctor or health care professional.*

 ### Yoga Exercise – Poses for constipation relief

Yoga is one of the best exercises you can do for your body health. It is not just ordinary exercise; it is a well-known science and uplifting practice.

- Yoga can help with many health issues and prevent many illnesses.
- Yoga exercises improve every single muscle in the body; it is very balanced and not harsh to the muscles and bones.
- **Yoga is for everyone** as everyone can optimize the yoga postures to his/her body capabilities.

Yoga can help a person to overcome constipation. The following asanas (yoga postures) have proven to be helpful in constipation relief. All of them strengthen abdominal muscles, intestine muscles, and abdominal organs. They encourage peristalses and generally assist digestion.

*Do not forget to supplement Yoga exercise with healthy eating habits, enough sleep and drinking plenty of water.*

103

### Kapalabhati – Yogic Abdominal Breathing Exercise

1. Sit comfortably on the small cushion on the floor, cross-legged, with your back straight and your head erected.
2. Take slow two deep breaths.
3. Inhale, then contract your abdominal muscles, pull your belly in and strongly and forcefully exhale.
4. Relax your abdominal muscles. Passive inhalation will take place as diaphragm moves back into the abdominal cavity. Do not inhale forcefully.
5. Repeat this pumping 20-30 times, then take three slow and deep breaths and start another round of pumping. Again take three deep breaths and do one more round of pumping.
6. Slowly and deeply inhale, then exhale completely, inhale fully and hold your breath for as long as you comfortably can.
7. Relax.

Breath is short, strong and rapid. Breathing is abdominal; bring the air just into your abdomen, not into your chest. With exhalation abdominal muscles contract, with inhalation abdominal muscles relax.

Between the thoracic cavity and the abdominal cavity is a muscular partition called Diaphragm. Diaphragm performs an important function in respiration, it moves down as the lungs expands and up as the lungs contracts. During this process it massages intestines and helps peristaltic action. Deep breathing and exercise increase peristalsis.

### The Half Plough Posture (Ardha Halasana)

1. Lie flat on your back, legs stretched, big toes and heels together, arms beside your side with the palms facing down.
2. Inhale, press the palms down and raise the left leg up slowly as high as you can with the knee straight and your back close to the floor as possible. The other leg is resting on the floor also straight.
3. As you exhale, bring the leg slowly down and repeat the process with the right leg.
4. Repeat the whole process three times or more.
5. With inhalation press the palms down and raise very slowly both legs up without bending the knees. Stay for few moments with your legs up, breathe comfortably.
6. With exhalation press the palms down again and very slowly bring both legs down to the floor. Relax as long as you want.
7. Repeat whole process three times or more.


### The Half Wind Relieving Pose (Ardha Pavanamuktasana)

1. Lie flat on your back, with your arms by your side
2. Bend your left knee and bring it towards your chest.
3. Wrap your hands around the left knee and slowly bring it a little bit closer to the chest.
4. Raise you head towards the knee and bring your chin towards the kneecap. Hold this posture for 10-30 seconds, breathe normally and then release.
5. Repeat with the right leg.
6. Repeat the whole process 4 times.

### The Wind Relieving Pose (Pavanamuktasana)

1. Lie flat on your back, with your arms by your side
2. Bend your both knees and bring them close to your chest.
3. Wrap your hands around your knees and bring then little bit closer to your chest.
4. Raise your head towards your knees and bring your chin towards the kneecaps. Hold for 10-30 seconds, breathe normally and then release.
5. Relax.
6. Repeat 3 times.

Those who suffer from any neck injuries should keep their head on the floor (or yoga mat).

### Shoulderstand (Sarvangasana)

1. Lie flat on your back, leg straight, feet together, arms beside your sides, palms down.
2. With inhalation raise both your legs up towards the ceiling until they are at the right angle to your torso.
3. Lift the pelvis and torso up (you may swing your legs over your head first to provide a counterweight for lifting up the pelvis and torso).
4. Bend the elbows and support your back with your hands. Rest on your shoulders, breathe normally. Adjust the posture by moving your hands towards your shoulder blades and lifting the legs and hips upward. Legs and torso should be straight and at a right angle to the floor (If you are beginner do not worry if your posture is straight or not as the posture will improve with your practise).

5. Hold the posture for 30 seconds to 3 minutes, breathe normally.

6. With exhalation lover your legs to a 45 degree angel over your head, place your arms back on the floor behind your back with palms facing down, and vertebra come down to the floor as slowly as possible. Relax and repeat the whole process 2 times.

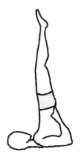

Do not practice Shoulderstand if you have any neck or shoulder injuries.

**Seated Forward Bend** *(Paschimothanasana)*

1. Sit down on the floor with your legs together and stretched, with the toes pointing back to the body.

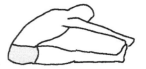

2. Inhale, raise your arms up over your head, and stretch your back upwards as much as you can.

3. While exhaling slowly bend forward, gaze on front of you, and reach for the toes. Keep your back and legs straight. Pull in the stomach.

4. If you cannot reach the toes, hold on to your ankles or your shins. Eventually gaze down on your legs.

5. Hold the posture, breathe deeply. With every exhale breadth slowly, try to come forward a little bit more.

6. Hold the posture from 20 second to 5 minutes (depends on your physical abilities).

7. Inhale, stretch the body forward and upward and slowly come back to the sitting posture with your arms rose up above your head. Relax the arms.
8. Repeat 2-3 times.

### Cobra Pose (Bhujangasana)

1. Lie face down on your belly with your body straight, your legs together, your forehead rests on your hands which are placed one on top of the other to make a pillow.
2. Lift your head a little bit, bring hands directly beneath the respective shoulders and place them flat on the floor, palms facing downward, rest your forehead on the floor.
3. With inhalation begin to roll slowly like a snake, raise your head up and back. Push your hands into the floor, raise your chest off the floor, and slowly arch your upper body up and back. Legs and hips stay on the floor, elbows stay slightly bent. Push shoulders down and back.
4. Make sure that your weigh is not just on your arms; your lower back should do most of the work. Hold the position for about 10 second to 1 minute. Breathe normally.
5. With exhalation roll slowly out of the posture, last lower your forehead on the floor.
6. Relax and repeat the whole process 2-3 times.

### The Half Locust

1. Lie face down on the floor on your stomach with your body straight, legs stretched, and your arms stretched by your sides.

2. Bring your arms underneath your body with your elbows as close to each other as possible. You can make fists from your hands or simply rest your palms facing down or up on the floor. Stretch your chin forward as far as you can and rest it on the floor or yoga mat. Gaze forward.

3. With inhalation raise your right leg off the floor as high as you can, do not twist your hips, do not bend your knee, and do not push into the floor with your left leg.

4. Hold this posture for about 5 to 30 seconds, breathe normally. With exhalation lower your right leg on the floor and repeat the same with your left leg.

5. Repeat on each side 2-3 times.

## The Locust (Shalabhasana)

1. Lie face down on the floor on your stomach with your body straight, legs stretched, and your arms stretched by your sides.

2. Bring your arms underneath your body with your elbows as close to each other as possible. You can make fists from your hands or simply rest your palms facing down or up on the floor. Stretch your chin forward as far as you can and rest it on the floor or yoga mat. Gaze forward.

3. With inhalation raise both your legs off the floor as high as you can, do not bend your knees. Hold the posture as long as you can, breathe normally.

4. With exhalation slowly lower your legs on the floor and rest as long as you want.

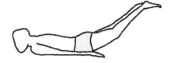

5.  Repeat whole process 3 times.

If you are yoga beginner you may find that you will not be able to raise your legs too high. Do not be disappointed. Once you practice you will be able to raise your legs higher and higher each time.

Beginners variation

1.  Lie face down on the floor on your stomach with your body straight, legs stretched, and with your arms stretched above your head.
2.  With inhalation raise your legs and your arms up, supporting your body on your abdomen. Gaze forward.
3.  Hold the posture for 10 to 30 seconds.
4.  Release with exhalation and repeat the whole process 3 times.

Do not practice The Half Locust or The Full Locust during pregnancy.

**The Bow (Dhanurasana)**

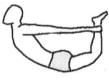

1.  Lie face down on your stomach with your body straight, legs stretched, and with your arms stretched by your sides, palms facing upwards. Your forehead is touching the ground.
2.  With exhalation bend your knees, reach back with both hands and catch hold of the respective ankles.
3.  With inhalation raise your head, chest and thighs off the floor, arch your body upwards.
4.  Hold the pose for 10 to 30 second, breathe normally. You may try to rock your body forward and backward.

110

5.  With exhalation release the pose. Relax and repeat whole process 3 times.

Do not practice The Bow during pregnancy.

### Half Spinal Twist (Ardha Matsyendrasana)

1.  Sit up on your heels.
2.  Drop the hips to the floor on the left of the hips.
3.  Place the right foot flat on the floor just on the outside of the left knee. The right foot is touching outside of the left knee. Keep the spine erect.
4.  Raise the right arm up, and then bring it to the floor behind the back. Raise the left arm up, and bring it over the right side of the right knee. With exhalation slowly twist right. Your left hand is holding your right ankle.
5.  Look over the right shoulder. As you exhale try to twist little bit more to your left.
6.  Hold for one minute, then release and repeat on the other side.
7.  Repeat the posture few times.

Beginners variation – instead of sitting on your heels sit up upright with legs together straight out in front of your body. Bend the right knee and bring the right foot just outside the left knee. Raise the right arm up and then bring it to the floor behind your back. Raise the left arm up and bring it over your right leg touching the right knee from outside. Twist right and look over your right shoulder. Your left hand is holding your right ankle. Hold for half a minute to one minute, release and repeat on the other side.

### Triangle Pose (Trikonasana)

1. Stand straight with your hands by your side and the feet wide apart.
2. Turn the left foot 90 degrees angle to the left.
3. As you inhale, raise the right arm up as much as you can, as you exhale bend your torso to your left.
4. Slide the left arm down your left leg to the left calf, the right arm is parallel to the floor now.
5. Do not turn your hips; legs and arms are straight, there should not be any weight on the lower arm, gaze straight in front of you or up to the ceiling.
6. Hold for 30 second, building up to 2 minutes, then release and repeat on the other side.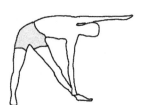
7. Repeat the posture 3 times.

### Diamond Pose (Supta Vajrasana)

1. Sit up on your heels.
2. Slide with your bum on the floor, left foot is resting beside the left hip and right foot is resting beside the right hip.
3. Bend backwards and lay flat down on your back. Use both hands to support yourself while lying down.
4. Fold the hands behind your head, close the eyes and focus on your breathing.
5. Retain the position for 30 seconds, building up to three minutes.
6. Return to sitting on your heels position.

Supta Vajrasana is not suitable for those who suffer from knee injuries, pain in the knee or hips, or lower back injuries.

## *Conclusion*

In this book, I have given you a lot of practical ways to get rid of constipation. I hope it has contributed to your health and wellbeing.

Congratulation to those who developed normal bowel functioning.

I have some final words for those who tried everything from this book but "nothing worked" yet or for those who have to take medication that cause constipation - use enemas (page 27) on a regular basis. It is simple to use, the whole process just takes a few minutes. Continue with a balanced and healthy diet. Keep taking supplements, drinking herbal teas, continue massaging your abdomen area, do your yoga exercises, etc. It is all good for you and sooner or later will contribute to your better bowel functioning.

# Glossary of Terms

**amino acids**   Amino acids are molecules critical to life, and have many functions in metabolism. They form proteins and function as chemical messengers and as intermediates in metabolism.

**amyloidosis**   Amyloidosis is a group of diseases that result from the abnormal deposition of a particular protein, called amyloid, in various tissues of the body.

**anaemia**   Anaemia is a condition caused by a lack of red blood cells or less than the normal quantity of hemoglobin in the blood.

**anaerobic bacteria**   Bacteria that do not live in the presence of oxygen. In humans, this type of bacteria is most commonly found in the gastrointestinal tract. It plays a role in conditions such as appendicitis, diverticulitis, and perforation of the bowel.

**anal fissures**   An anal fissure is a crack or tear in the skin of the anal canal.

**aneurysm**   Aneurysm is a blood-filled balloon-like bulge of a blood vessel.

**anus**   Excretory opening at the end of the alimentary canal.

**appendicitis**   Appendicitis is a condition characterized by inflammation of the appendix.

**arthritis**   Arthritis is a group of conditions involving damage to the joints of the body.

**atherosclerosis**   Atherosclerosis is a condition in which an artery wall thickens as the result of a build-up of fatty materials such as cholesterol.

**atonic colon**   Lack of normal muscle tone or strength in the colon.

**atonic dyspepsia**   Dyspepsia with impaired tone in the muscular walls of the stomach.

**atony of the urinary bladder**   A large dilated urinary bladder that fails to empty properly.

**Ayurvedic medicine**    Ayurvedic medicine is a system of traditional medicine native to the Indian subcontinent and practiced in other parts of the world as a form of alternative medicine.

**bolus**    Bolus is a ball-shaped mass moving through the digestive tract.

**bronchitis**    Bronchitis is inflammation of the mucous membranes of the bronchi, the airways that carry airflow from the trachea into the lungs.

**ceacum**    The caecum is a pouch, connecting the ileum with the ascending colon of the large intestine.

**casein**    Casein is the predominant phosphoprotein that accounts for nearly 20% of proteins in cow milk and cheese.

**catarrh**    Catarrh is a disorder of inflammation of the mucous membranes.

**celiac disease**    Coeliac disease is an autoimmune disorder of the small intestine.

**cellulose**    Cellulose is the structural component of the primary cell wall of green plants, many forms of algae and the oomycetes.

**colitis**    Colitis is an inflammation of the colon.

**colostomy**    Colostomy is a surgical construction of an artificial excretory opening from the colon.

**constipation    Constipation** refers to bowel movements that are infrequent and hard to pass.

**convulsions**    A convulsion is a medical condition where body muscles contract and relax rapidly and repeatedly, resulting in an uncontrolled shaking of the body.

**coronary heart disease**    Coronary heart disease refers to the failure of coronary circulation to supply adequate circulation to cardiac muscle and surrounding tissue.

**dandruff**    Dandruff is the shedding of dead skin cells from the scalp.

**dental abscesses**   A dental abscess is pus enclosed in the tissues of the jaw bone at the tip of an infected tooth.

**diarrhoea**   Frequent and watery bowel movements.

**diverticulitis**   Digestive disease particularly found in the large intestine. Diverticulitis develops from diverticulosis, which involves the formation of pouches (diverticula) on the outside of the colon. Diverticulitis results if one of these diverticula becomes inflamed.

**dropsy**   Dropsy is an abnormal accumulation of fluid beneath the skin or in one or more cavities of the body.

**dysentery**   Dysentery is an inflammatory disorder of the intestine, especially of the colon, that results in severe diarrhoea containing mucus and/or blood in the feces with fever and abdominal pain.

**dyspepsia**   Dyspepsia is a medical condition characterized by chronic or recurrent pain in the upper abdomen, upper abdominal fullness and feeling full earlier than expected when eating.[2] It can be accompanied by bloating, belching, nausea, or heartburn.

**enteritis**   inflammation of the small intestine most commonly caused by the ingestion of substances contaminated with pathogenic microorganisms.

**fatty acids**   Fatty acids are the molecules making up fats and oils and are released when oils and fats are broken down in the digestive system. They provide a source of energy.

**fibre**   Fibre is the indigestible carbohydrate found in fruit, vegetables, grain and nuts.

**fibroids**   Fibroids are common, benign tumors of smooth muscle in the uterus (womb).

**flatulence**   The presence of excessive gas in the digestive tract.

**flavonoids**   Flavonoids are polyphenol antioxidants found naturally in plants. They are beneficial to the human body when consumed in the form of fruits and vegetables.

**folate**   A naturally occurring member of the B vitamin family. It is found in high concentrations in dark green vegetables and the legumes.

**folic acid**   The synthetic folate is called folic acid.

**furunculosis**   A condition in which the patient suffers from recurrent episodes of boils.

**gastritis**   Gastritis is an inflammation of the lining of the stomach.

**gliadin**   Gliadin is a glycoprotein present in wheat and several other cereals.

**gluten**   Gluten (from Latin *gluten* "glue") is the composite of two proteins called *gliadin* and *glutenin*.

**glutenin**   Glutenin is a simple protein found in wheat.

**gout**   Gout is a medical condition characterized by recurrent attacks of acute inflammatory arthritis.

**heart palpitations**   Abnormality of heartbeat that causes a conscious awareness of its beating.

**hemicellulose**   Any of several polysaccharides that are more complex than a sugar and less complex than cellulose, found in plant cell walls

**hypocalcaemia**   Hypocalcaemia is the presence of low serum calcium levels in the blood.

**hypoproteinaemia**   Hypoproteinaemia is a condition where there is an abnormally low level of protein in the blood.

**irritable bowel syndrome**   Gastrointestinal disorder involving an abnormal condition of gut contractions characterized by abdominal pain, bloating, mucous in stools, and irregular bowel habits with alternating constipation and diarrhea.

**insomnia**   An inability to sleep; chronic sleeplessness.

**jaundice**   Jaundice is a yellowish pigmentation of the skin, the whites of the eyes, and other mucous membranes caused by increased levels of bilirubin in the blood.

**lactose**   Lactose is a sugar that is found in milk.

**laryngitis**   Laryngitis is an inflammation of the larynx, the portion of the respiratory tract.

**lecithin**  An antioxidant, emulsifier, and dietary supplement used to lower cholesterol, to provide cardiovascular support, to treat liver and kidney conditions, and to aid in the treatment of some central nervous system disorders.

**lethargy**  A state of sluggishness, inactivity, and apathy.

**lignin**  A complex polymer that binds to cellulose fibers and hardens and strengthens the cell walls of plants.

**lupus**  Connective tissue disorder.

**lutein**  Lutein is a one of naturally-occurring carotenoids.

**malabsorption**  Malabsorption is abnormality in absorption of food nutrients across the gastrointestinal tract.

**meningitis**  Meningitis is inflammation of the protective membranes covering the brain and spinal cord.

**microvilli**  Tiny hairlike folds that extend from the surface of many absorptive or secretory cells.

**mono-unsaturated fats**  Mono-unsaturated fat is a type of fatty acid that can lower blood cholesterol levels.

**mucus**  Mucus is a slippery secretion produced by, and covering, mucous membranes.

**multiple sclerosis**  Multiple sclerosis is a nervous system disease that affects the brain and spinal cord.

**myasthenia gravis**  Myasthenia gravis is an autoimmune neuromuscular disease leading to fluctuating muscle weakness and fatiguability.

**nausea**  Nausea is a sensation of unease and discomfort in the upper stomach with an urge to vomit.

**neuralgia**  Neuralgia is the medical term used to describe nerve pain.

**neuritis**  Neuritis is a general term for inflammation of a nerve[4] or the general inflammation of the portion of the nervous system.

**oesophagus**  The oesophagus is a muscular tube in the chest that connects the mouth and throat to the stomach.

**osteoporosis**   Osteoporosis is a disease of bones characterized by a decrease in the density of bone, decreasing its strength and resulting in fragile bones.

**pancreatitis**   Pancreatitis is inflammation of the pancreas.

**pectin**   Pectin is a structural heteropolysaccharide found in the cell walls of plants.

**pepsin**   A digestive enzyme found in gastric juice.

**peristalsis**   Peristalsis is the wave-like contractions that move food along the digestive tract.

**peritonitis**   Peritonitis is an inflammation of the peritoneum, the serous membrane that lines part of the abdominal cavity and viscera.

**pernicious anaemia**   Pernicious anaemia is a blood disorder caused by inadequate vitamin B12 in the blood.

**Pharynx**   The **pharynx** is a part of the digestive tube placed behind the nasal cavities, mouth, and larynx.

**phytic acid**   **Phytic acid** is the principal storage form of phosphorus in many plant tissues, especially bran and seeds.

**poly-unsaturated fats**   polyunsaturated fatty acid, are fatty acids that have more than one double-bonded (unsaturated) carbon in the molecule. It is an essential element in our diet.

**probiotic**   Probiotics are beneficial microorganisms found in the human digestive system.

**Prolapse**   The falling, sinking, or sliding of an organ from its normal location in the body.

**proteolytic enzyme**   Proteolytic enzyme (protease) help with digestion of the proteins in food.

**psoriasis**   Psoriasis is a chronic, autoimmune disease that appears on the skin.

**Raynaud's disease**   Raynaud's disease is a disorder causing discoloration of the fingers, toes, and occasionally other areas.

**rectum**   The rectum is the final straight portion of the large intestine.

**rheumatoid arthritis**   Rheumatoid arthritis is a chronic, inflammatory disorder that may affect many tissues and organs, but principally attacks synovial joints.

**scabies**   Scabies is a contagious ectoparasitic skin infection characterized by superficial burrows and intense itching.

**sciatica**   Pain along the sciatic nerve usually caused by a herniated disk of the lumbar region of the spine.

**scleroderma**   Scleroderma is a chronic systemic autoimmune disease characterized by thickening and hardening of the skin.

**scrapes**   Scrapes are skin wounds that rub or tear off skin.

**sigmoid**   The sigmoid is the part of the colon after the descending colon and before the rectum.

**sterol**   Sterols are an important class of organic molecules which occur naturally in plants, animals, and fungi.

**Tamari**   Tamari is the "original" Japanese soy sauce, made with more soybeans than ordinary soy sauce.

**thrombosed haemorrhoid**   External haemorrhoid with the vein ruptures and/or a blood clot.

**typhoid**   Typhoid is a fever transmitted by the ingestion of food or water contaminated with the feces, which contain the bacterium Salmonella typhi.

**uraemia**   A toxic condition resulting from the accumulation of waste products normally excreted in the urine, in the blood.

**vegetable mucilage**   A gelatinous substance obtained from certain plants.

**villi**   Villi are tiny, finger-like projections that are approximately 0.5-1mm in length and cover the lining of the small intestine.

**Xylitol**   Xylitol is a sweetener used as a naturally occurring sugar substitute.

CPSIA information can be obtained at www.ICGtesting.com
Printed in the USA
BVOW06s1826170816

459340BV00022B/137/P